HUGH GIVES YOU:™

4 FANTASTIC FITNESS/FAT LOSS METHODS TO USE!

With inspiring tips, facts, stats, and pics.

Hugh Esling

Produced by:

FriesenPress

Suite 300 – 852 Fort Street
Victoria, BC, Canada V8W 1H8

www.friesenpress.com

Distributed to the trade by The Ingram Book Company

Table of Contents

Acknowledgements

Thanks Kerry, for suggesting I write a book on losing weight and getting fit.

And thank you Kaitlin, for pointing out in the first place that I was "getting pretty big."

And a final thanks to Christopher for providing me with so many ideas and much encouragement along the way.

Disclaimer

The information provided in this book is designed to provide helpful information on the subjects discussed. This information and advice written or made available through this book is not intended to replace the services of a physician or a health care or fitness professional. This book is not meant to be used, nor should it be used, to diagnose or treat any medical condition. For diagnosis or treatment of any medical problem, consult your own physician. Each individual's results may vary based upon their circumstances and the individual's specific situation. There are no guarantees as to outcomes. My personal methods of weight loss and firming up, while solely created, tested, and reported by myself, are not intended to convey any warranty, either express or implied, as to outcomes, promises, or benefits.

The author and publisher make no representation or warranties with respect to the accuracy, applicability, or completeness of the contents of this book. The information contained in this book is strictly for informational purposes. References are provided for informational purposes only and do not constitute endorsement of any websites or other sources. Therefore, if you apply the ideas contained in this book, you are accepting full responsibility for your actions.

About The Author

I was born at a very early age. By grade one I had been expelled, in grade two I had the school in a riot, in grade three I got the strap just for being me, and in grade six I made the news in one, for sure, major Toronto paper, the now defunct Toronto Telegram, and had the police, firefighters, Mom, Dad, and pretty well everyone else shocked and pissed with my storm sewer tours.

Then I became a guinea pig and turned my attention to weight gains, losses and fitness personal bests. And things started to get crazy.

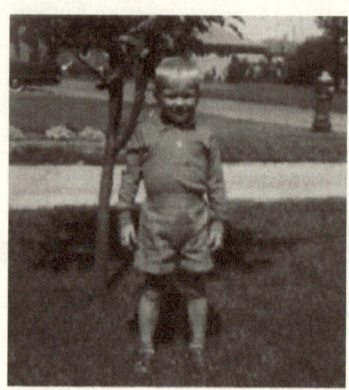

Part One

On human nature: Don't get lost in the snakes and ladders of self destructive tendencies or fall through the trap doors of self satisfaction, procrastination, and distraction.

Chapter 1
Introduction and method one

Do you want to lose lots of fat? Do you want to get really fit? You've come to the right place. The two parts of this book will inspire you to do either, or both. Let's be clear. Each of us has a unique set of circumstances in our quest to be the absolute best we can be physically.

I am like so many of you. I got very fat. I wanted to get fit.

But for this book I got fat four times, the last two times on purpose.

As an analyst (and a guinea pig) I wanted to provide you with four completely different methods to lose fat and attain fitness personal bests.

These methods, which took nine years from inception to completion, and other great fitness tips and strategies, form part one of the book.

There is no one magic formula for weight loss. If you want to lose weight big-time and firm up while smoking, drinking, and eating what you want, (Method 1) you can do it. If you want to lose weight by watching what you eat and working out with a physical fitness instructor, (Method 2) you can do it. If you want to lose weight *very* quickly and save a bundle on food costs, (Method 3) you can do it. If you want to lose weight sanely and gradually, without stepping on a scale, and keep that weight off for the rest of your life (Method 4) —you can do that too.

One or more of these methods may be ideal for you. The *proof* of each method's success is backed up by *clear* pictures of progress, readily understandable exercise and fat loss explanations, and at-a-glance, easy-to-read, tables outlining average *daily* results in pounds/kilograms dropped.

The second part, to further inspire you, highlights fantastic fitness exploits. We will marvel at individuals, sports, and activities. Part two will also, albeit in a dramatically different way, motivate you to avoid, or change, certain behaviors. We will learn not only of examples of individual sloth but of incredible—true—examples in social, legal, and political overreach—locally, nationally, and globally—in deciding, if we, *or our children, or parents*, are too fat.

The pieces for the second part were written over the past few years. Efforts have been made to update them, where possible and applicable, to just before this book went to print.

I can't stress enough how clearly I wanted to show you (it's the analyst in me coming out again) that no matter what your situation is today, you can take any one of these methods, or even parts of each, to shape up and slim down.

And live by this:

Your fitness goals should be concise. A workout should contain no unnecessary meanderings for the same reason a paragraph should contain no unnecessary sentences and a recipe no unnecessary ingredients. Have specific targets and make every motion count.

The book's end serves up obesity myths, gives you (again, for they are provided in Table 1) not only the constants I used through all four methods to drop fat and get buff, but also gives you *the* tip to be your absolute best physically.

Throughout the book you have fact, not fiction, empiricism, not euphemism. You are serious about your goals. You have serious answers here, sprinkled with mirth as I retell all the trials and tribulations along the way that turned to triumph.

Triumph that can be yours.

Table 1: The four methods I used in detail, with time taken, and weight lost

Method	1	2	3	4
Smoking	Y	N	N	N
Alcohol	Y	N	N	N**
Junk food	Y	N	N	N
Walking	Y	Y	Y	Y
Elliptical	Y	Y	Y	Y
Weight training	Y	Y	Y	Y
Tracking progress	Y	Y	Y	Y
Weigh ins – scale	Y	Y	Y	N
Fitness trainer	N	Y	N	N
Pounds lost	72	37*	36	35*
Time taken	3 years	72 days	50 days	215 days
Average pounds lost per day	0.066	0.514	0.72	.0163
Average grams lost per day	29.94	233.15	326.59	73.94

* For Method 2 the total lost was 61 pounds (27 kg), in just under 6 months (173 days), with the last 24 pounds coming off after my sessions with my trainer ended. The average

pounds, therefore, lost per day with Method 2 before and after my fitness trainer was 61 pounds/173 days = 0.353 lost per day (grams 160.12 day.)

* For Method 4 the 35 pounds dropped happened between July 1, 2012 and January 31, 2013. But Method 4, with my final picture taken just before this book went to print, officially ended June 30, 2013. ** Unofficially I will be thriving by Method 4 for the rest of my life, saving for the occasional drink with friends. It is, by far, the easiest to maintain for diet, yet improve for fitness levels, of all the four methods.

Numbers don't lie. Notice Methods 2, 3, and 4 resulted in much greater average pounds/grams loss per day, as compared with Method 1. Why? No junk food, alcohol, or cigarettes. The defense rests…

Why Method 1? Because I Was One Couch Potato…

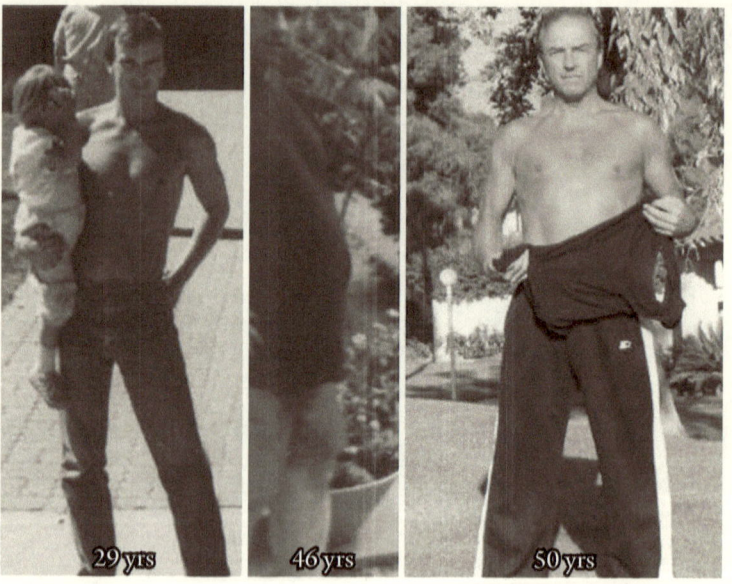

The wheezing finally did me in. When I breathed at all, I wheezed. My goal, when I could struggle off the couch, was to hunt around in the fridge. I was a 46-inch (117centimeter) "waisted" (and wasted), 217 pound (98 kilogram) 47-year-old guy. I was 46 when the middle blimp picture was taken, but I was just as pitiful when I started one year later with Method 1.

I had, it is clear, fattened up since about 30. It happened, as it does to most of us I suspect, innocently enough. Work, family, and friends, the latter the kind that like to imbibe and gab, took precedence over regular exercise, or any sporting pastimes. Nothing criminal here, but definitely nothing exemplary either as a lifestyle choice.

But this wheeze, after my third "power nap" of the day, instilled an emotion in me I had not felt since I was a tyke trying to make the hockey team: desperation. I was desperate to stop the wheezing, and I suddenly remembered that I hadn't been prone to gasping when I was in good shape. So it was time to shape up—or ship out.

You can't blame me for loving the couch. Everyone loves a comfy sofa and couch potato surfing, hour after hour, is good for the soul and spirit—so long as life's chores are somewhat attended, or at least kept in check. But my loafing had passed the moderate stage years (a decade?) back. The only reason I did not have bed sores was that I was too lazy and tuckered out to crash on a bed, preferring the couch.

But we all know that a couch, while good for the soul, does nothing positive for the body. A life lounged is not a life lived.

I did not need to buy a "Lazy Boy." I had become one.

The wheeze had to go. And thus the couch. And all the sloth, and all the slouch.

Desperation is a real tonic, a pick-me-up if you will. It enabled me to see clearly and decide to start a weight training program and go back to the health club I had deserted, save for showers and shaving, eons ago.

Perhaps desperation can be an enlightenment for you too, one that will help you eschew the fright and embrace the fight. The fight to get fit.

Before I get into specifics, let us step back and look at two factors that usually hover around any goals, whether they are physical, educational, or vocational: hope and inspiration.

How to make hope work for you

How does hope fit into the exercise equation? Is it a useless emotion, or worse, an illusion that acts as an impediment? Or is it an emotional engine that spurs one on to health heights previously unimagined?

Not to be too dramatic, but on a bad day when everything goes wrong, sometimes hope is the small installment of salvation that keeps us going, envisioning a better tomorrow. But if it is a torch with no athlete, it is worse than nothing because it gives the impression of accomplishment with no reality underneath.

Benjamin Franklin said: "He that lives upon hope will die fasting."

Let no exercise program, no fitness regimen, no clean living protocol be held hostage by hope. Yet always carry hope as a companion on your journey in self-improvement for it is the basket in which all good and great dreams are carried.

Chapter 2
Inspiration and your fitness plan

Method One: Focus on fitness, not diet or other lifestyle issues

My fight to get fit, specifically and coincidentally, began on the day that US Vice President Dick Cheney checked into George Washington University Hospital because he was short of breath. On that same Saturday, November 13, 2004, a couple of minutes before 7:43 PM, afflicted by wheezing, I picked up my solitary five pound dumbbell and did 13 arm "movements."

I logged my efforts into a Microsoft Access database because I tracked nearly everything I do for work in there (and this was certainly work). I used the word "movements" because I did not want to get bogged down in specifying what type of arm exercise I was doing. I wanted to track my exertions while avoiding a cumbersome process. Between that date and Wednesday, February 9, 2005—the date I first dared to work out again at my health club, I did *all* arm movements with the dumbbell slowly and methodically. I was acutely aware that weight training, even with a puny five-pound dumbbell, could result in pain or injury, both of which I intended to avoid scrupulously because I wanted nothing to set me back.

I had started. And I finished that evening's efforts around 11:20 PM.

I converted the data tracked in Access into an Excel Table:

Task	Reps	Time	Date	With	Comments
Exercise	13	7:43:07 PM	11/13/2004	Arms	13 Movements with Dumbbell
Exercise	16	8:09:50 PM	11/13/2004	Arms	16 Movements with Dumbbell (Overheads)
Exercise	10	9:19:21 PM	11/13/2004	Arms	10 Movements with Dumbbell (Twisting and Outward Motion) Now some more...
Exercise	14	10:00:48 PM	11/13/2004	Arms	14 Movements with Dumbbell (Left Arm Overhead Raises)
Exercise	11	10:18:59 PM	11/13/2004	Arms	11 Movements with Dumbbell (Right Arm Overhead Raises)
Exercise	9	10:26:01 PM	11/13/2004	Arms	9 Movements with Dumbbell (Right Arm Wrist Curls)
Exercise	15	10:57:13 PM	11/13/2004	Arms	15 Movements with Dumbbells (Straight out Both Arms)
Exercise	11	11:20:39 PM	11/13/2004	Arms	11 Movements with Dumbbell (Left Arm Overhead Raises)
Sum	99				

You may well wonder, after looking at the comments field on the far right, why I consider this a non-cumbersome means of tracking progress. In Access, and now fortunately in Excel also, comments can be set to repeat themselves, once entered into a table. I was glad to have an accurate account of my actions without ever typing a given comment again. It would appear, in Access in highlights, and/or from a pull down box, and in Excel it would appear in highlights.

The Time and Date fields in Access are auto-data populated when typing begins in either the Task, Reps, With, or Comments field. The Task and With fields, like the Comments field, repeat the typed words thereafter, having being entered once into each. Indeed, the only field where typing was always necessary was the Reps field. Given that it was a number field, it took very little typing, or data entry, at all. Of course, any system, has to work for you. If you don't want to enter information in all the fields, don't. You can, of course, choose your own short forms for words or phrases.

No matter how you wish to chart your fitness path, you *should* write your results down, in one form or another. Keeping track "in your head" just won't cut it. Noting your good works in print commits you by the very act of inscribing it. I'll expand upon tracking progress later.

And I must 'fess up now. While using this first method, I did not govern what, when, why, or where I ate. I figured that just changing my life to add exercise was a big enough adjustment. I also did not attempt to cut back on my minimum two to three packs of cigarettes per week, nor did I tamper with tippling dark rum (any brand, love them all). Coming from Canada where ice hockey rules, I had heard of many NHL stars, like Guy Lafleur and Denis Savard, who smoked during their best years on ice. I hoped that daily exercise might prove a catalyst to curb my puffing and swilling. (I was a social smoker but I sure wasn't social toward it. I hated it every time I inhaled all that gunk.)

I did cut back on both drinking and smoking, not only because it's hard to partake while on an elliptical at a health club but because I just didn't feel the urge so often. As I began to feel better physically and mentally, I did not need these crutches for whatever was previously missing in my life. Life just felt a whole lot better without smoking and drinking.

Being an analyst by profession, I knew that the fat I had put on over 15-plus years would take two to three years to come off if I focused strictly on exercise and not diet at all. I was fine with that. I was not looking for an overnight miracle cure or magical method because, frankly, anything that sounds too good to be true, *is* too good to be true. I reasoned that prudence—and patience—would see me through.

Patience, however, given our wired world, our insatiable attitudes seeking instant gratification, and our general operating modes of hurry up harder, is in short supply. But patience is much more than a virtue, it's a necessity if one wants to lose weight and firm up without getting frustrated. Or injured. Or both.

It's easy to see why patience is rarer than an anorexics' Las Vegas hotel buffet. Look around: people stomp their feet and fume if they have to wait more than five minutes for their coffee perk-me-up—the latter is the fuel to insure a totally "productive" day. A news story of geopolitical global import, or of a tawdry scandal, lasts 15 minutes in the media. Then we need a new fix to keep us transfixed for the next 15 minutes while we dart past a slow-poke driver in the left lane so we can swerve in front of him and "win" by getting to wait five seconds longer than him at the next red light.

Slowing down and being methodical is not a crime against humanity. Painstakingly plotting your fitness program no more makes you a loafer than does taking the extra time at work to make that report "just so." On the contrary, it'll make you a winner. But the deadlines you set for weight loss and exercising must be firm yet flexible to take into account the reality of changing circumstances. If your plans are thrown off target you must not freak but rather be patient and simply state that your goals, while inviolate, will not be violated if they take a little longer to realize. Speed junkies are often flunkies. The quick fix is usually a trick.

Method 1 was no quick fix, that's for sure. It was a slow steady Eddie program and process that took 3 years to chop off the 72 pounds. Here's what I did and did not do.

Table 2: Using Method 1 for 3 years

Method	1
Smoking	Y
Alcohol	Y
Junk food	Y
Walking	Y
Elliptical	Y
Weight training	Y
Tracking progress	Y
Weigh ins- scale	Y
Fitness trainer	N
Pounds lost	72
Time taken	3 years
Average pounds lost per day	0.066
Average grams lost per day	29.94

Where to look for inspiration?

A drizzly afternoon, a stormy, lightning-filled evening, a snowy morning, all can inspire athletic accomplishment if you take a "me against the elements" viewpoint. But don't go off the deep end here: don't battle Mother Nature in her own back-yard. Stick your tongue out at her as you stick to your weights and walking from the warm, comfy confines of your health club.

And what of a sunny, cloudless, robin-egg-blue-sky color day? Does that not gal-vanize one to exercise energetically? If you keep track of your fitness personal bests, and these will be discussed later in the book, take charge and take heart knowing that the workout to come will see you hit new heights in speeds met, distances topped, amounts lifted, or repetitions done.

For those of us that do workout on our own, or go to fitness classes of any type, we know that exercise, besides improving our physical health, breeds such wonderful attributes of character, curiosity, and competition, prudence, power, and progress.

This inspiring Chinese proverb says it all about improving one's being through exercise: "The best time to plant a tree was 20 years ago. The second best time is now."

Chapter 3
Tracking fitness program progress

Tracking progress is essential to your success in losing weight and firming up. Why? As mentioned, the act of recording adds solemnity and seriousness to your pursuits. It makes it harder to fool yourself about what you are doing. Most of us, for many reasons, abhor the idea of tracking progress.

That's silly.

Iterations don't have to be like homilies of biblical proportions. They can be short, succinct, and sweet.

Here are the usual methods of tracking progress.

1. Memory.

2. Written record.

3. Database, table, or some type of spreadsheet record.

4. Fitness computer/phone applications.

Now, let us consider the value of each method:

Memory.

Memory is elusive: it is a newt, a salamander, the squishiest method for recall, and the likeliest to slink, sink, and shrivel under scrutiny.

Why is memory so haphazard? Because largely, memory is composed of (see A-E below). F) Totally accurate, honest memory does not appear here, nor is it discussed, because it is so rare that nobody has experienced it, nor in fact knows anyone who comes close to exhibiting it. But A-D, we've surely all seen and shown... and as for E) well, that's a special, sordid case.

A. Faulty memory.

B. Negligent memory.

C. Anecdotal memory.

D. Willful "BS" memory.

E. Lance Armstrong memory.

A) Faulty memory is mistaken memory. You assumed you forgot to do the wash on Wednesday but you are wrong; you forgot to do the wash on Monday, Tuesday, *and* Wednesday. Happens all the time, don't feel bad about it, move on. In training, this would occur when you believed, for example, you bench pressed 60 pounds in five repetitions whereas you actually did 50 pounds four times.

This is quite common; nothing to be alarmed about, other than you got your facts wrong.

B) Negligent memory is just that, negligent. You completely forgot that Saturday's workout session was forsaken as you were too busy drowning the kids' budgies, because they would not shut up. (The budgies, not the kids.) Negligent memory is worse than faulty memory, even for budgies. Negligent memory, with respect to training, is forgetting you have not worked out in a month and pretending, or fooling yourself, that you are only in a three-day detraining period (and not a month) thereby putting yourself on the shelf.

C) Anecdotal memory is downright fun. Remember the time—Wasn't that a scream?, Could you believe it when?—these are typical introductions to yarns and tall tales spun from anecdotal memory. You look to your past and apply this memory to recalling those peak physical periods and exploits. It has absolutely nothing to do with aiding your conditioning program of today. Anecdotal memory is a hoary historical record, embellished to relish.

D) Willful "BS" memory is when you make-believe a hash of a rehash of your past. This plays out as a lie to a prospect, a priest, a police officer, a palm reader, a pawn broker.

Simply recalling balderdash and bunk, then looming these into lies, distortions, and other disingenuous prevarications has no place in your training. You may talk up a storm of your tautness and strength as you remember and retell past acts, but if *you look like* a sack of gummy bears…

"BS" offers no benefit, if you do not count the derision from those forced to listen to your fibs.

E) Lance Armstrong memory is by far the worst type of memory to have, not so much because it is built on a huge house of lies but because it is an edifice of execrable maliciousness: smearing and threatening others who dare question its veracity.

Lance Armstrong memory is mendacious, governed as it is by the almighty dollar. Companies that sponsored Armstrong might have expected him to blow back against charges of doping. Whether they did, or did not, he certainly did.

Lance Armstrong memory is manipulative. Instead of serving the blank slate of reality, it serves the greasy spoon of media and consumer opinion.

Okay, poking fun at memory aside, let's look at the more well known and realistic methods of noting your notables.

Written record.

You may record your doings in a diary or journal, using both numerical and comments fields.

There is nothing wrong with this method; it certainly beats our five types of memory above, but recalling and and reporting upon your exploits is easier with system 3).

Database, table, or some type of spreadsheet record.

Two common software programs with database capabilities are MS Excel and MS Access.

A database can compile one table. For your fitness program a single table should work just fine. A table is filled with vertical—columns and horizontal rows of information. In Excel, columns are identified by letters, rows by numbers.

The big advantages over a written record are:

A. The copy paste function and

B. Automatic mathematical functions like additions, counts,
averages and percentages, to name but a few.

I developed a customized database in MS Access specific to my exercises that allows exercise words and phrases to be available in pop-up menus. Recording, rather than in a few minutes by typing the desired word or phrase , is as quick as a click. Less work in recording your sessions is crucial; most of us find this aspect of an exercise program a total drag and drop it, rationalizing the workout is the key. (In Excel, this feature of automatic data fill for a first-time data entry, is now also featured.)

You may argue that the workout is the real deal. It is true, but without working out you are nowhere without concrete tangible records of goals, and the recording of work to achieve those goals, you are more than likely setting yourself up to fall short. You'll still be lost. Writing, data entry, or computer/phone apps all serve to make permanent your performance production. They have the power of public oath. It is much harder to stomp all over your regimen if you've taken some time to tally and total your sessions.

My system is as simple as can be.

The categories are basic. You can certainly have many categories, it is a personal choice obviously, but these four have brought me success and take but seconds to record them.

Miles,

Arms,

Legs,

Sit-ups.

These are the backbone of my workouts and consequent analysis.

Repetitions, amounts, and commentary, all buttressed by time and date data, serve as the statistical fodder for filtering and sorting.

Fitness computer/phone applications.

While I don't use current apps, there's no reason for you not to. Check out the array of fitness, diet, health, and medical apps. Their pictures, videos, workout menus, maps, and instructions will school and tool you in Yoga, Pilates, musculature impact, Body Mass Index indications, running routes, you name it – they have it. Many cost three dollars or less. There is no excuse not to use what works for you.

Or you can use the perfectly suitable time-tested method of check marking a day on the wall or fridge calendar. Takes a second but tells you everything you need to know: "Yup, I was in the game, worked out today. Hooray."

Chapter 4
Weight training tips

Speaking of hope, here are some weight training tips that might work for you.

- Do visualize your ideal body.

- Do not stop visualizing it.

- Do exhale on exertions.

- Do not rush repetitions.

- Do emphasize form.

- Do not lean or list.

- Do focus on the muscles worked.

- Do not grunt, groan, or moan unless near collapse.

- Do ask for a spotter.

- Do not injure yourself.

- Do realize Rome was not built in a day.

- Do not expect visible changes until three weeks have passed after starting weight training.

- Do expect boredom unless you change your routine.

- Do not sit down in the weight room: you'll burn more calories standing.

- Do drink water.

- Do not fret if weight loss is slow to arrive, it can be capricious, unpredictable, and inexplicable. (Although Method 3 definitely debunks this!)

- Do avoid not exercising three days in a row, for de-training sets in.

- Do not rue the past, or fret of the future, but be in the now and concentrate.

- Do try to have fun.

- Do not sneer at the adage: "Every little bit helps."

- Do remember the above and don't you forget it.

And don't forget these fundamentals and facts either. Consider that the glass is already half full. Then you have three big advantages when beginning a fitness program from an overweight start.

You can set the tone and pace.

Rest assured, you don't have to worry about impressing anybody.

You get to pick the activities and exercises you like.

You do, however, have to do the actual work. There are no shortcuts, sorry. But don't overdo things. Listen to your body. At the first sign of strain or pain that doesn't feel quite right, stop, surmise, decide. Continue or cease, or ease back on the elbow grease? And make sure you take one day off per week from your regimen. Allow your body to rest and recuperate. The slow and steady approach to shedding fat is probably best: instead of trying to lose a pound a day, aim, perhaps, to lop off two pounds (.9 kilograms) per month. It seems a tad conservative, but annually it adds to subtract 24 pounds (10.88 kilograms), not a bad feat at that.

I personally also made a conscious decision owing to the size of my belly and the impossibility of doing proper sit ups, to work on my abdomen muscles later, once my curvature was approaching flatter proportions. Read up on everything, and adopt and adapt what makes sense to you in terms of risk and reward. Be prepared for peaks and plateaus, they are normal in the ebbs and flows of improving your condition. And though you may hate weight training, done properly and judiciously, your body will dig it.

Chapter 5
Timely fitness tips

Many of us do not like the gym or health club scene, and many more of us do not have a lot of spare time for exercise. What can be done to make sure you get in your fitness fix that fits?

Well, a workout of 20 minutes, although briefer than ideally desired, can make the grade with your fitness and timetable goals.

In other words, you could have 10 minutes for cardio and 10 minutes for weights. Optimally both parts would net the best results if you followed them intensely but if you are just starting out again, do not go intense but go slow and easy, and get that 20 minute workout chalked up on the big board. Over the year these 20 minute workouts add up to calories burned, fat dropped, and muscle packed on. If, until now, you have skipped a session because you thought 20 or 30 minutes would not be enough time, think again. Some exercise is always better than none.

You can always say you have little time. But you want the biggest bang for your buck. What should be cut back, cardio or weight training? In my opinion, the cardio.

Why? Weights take 10 minutes if done with rigor and resolve. If you keep the cardio and forgo the weights, yes you can run your face off, and yes you'll lose "X" amount of calories every mile, but that'll take you 20 to 40 minutes, and you might still be flabby.

In a January a few years ago, I had been averaging five miles (8.04 kilometers) per day on the elliptical. But it was then May and I had to clean up my house before the dust bunnies bloomed out of control. I had to get all my junk into piles so it could be taken away. I needed extra time. I threw the five miles per day out the window, did a mile (1.6 kilometers) a day instead, and upped my weight training intensity. The junk is pretty well gone, I'm taming the dust bunnies, and I didn't gain any weight. The weight work by day has me burning extra calories at night whilst dreaming of finding elusive, threatening dust bunnies. Not too shabby.

So trust in your exercise plans. Don't get lost in the snakes and ladders of self destructive tendencies or fall through the trap doors of self satisfaction, procrastination, and distraction. You can control, limit or mitigate these false flags with trust in yourself and the belief that you are on the right path. If you don't have faith in yourself, who will?

If you want to meet your fat-loss targets you must scrap the usual, normal, customary, and habitual. You will have to change your outlook, for obviously it has not been to great benefit so far, and this change in attitude and approach can be a freak out.

Yes this job, this task of shedding fat and shaping up, may be new and strange, but that fact need not immobilize you. This battle of the bulge can be won if you mentally tear down the ramparts of ingrained ways. So don't be rigid and frigid, cold, and unyielding with a dogmatic attitude in your approach to getting fit. These attitudes are not only constraining, they carry the seeds of failure.

And beware of claustrophobia. Say what? Yes, claustrophobia can occur if you are a slave to a do-or-die mentality that each goal must be met.

Nuts to that. If you do not make a daily, weekly, or monthly target, don't paint yourself into a corner and amplify your personal miss with a broad-brush, failure complex. Do not let logical thought succumb to guilt over an unmet opportunity. Keep a positive attitude despite temporary inadequacy.

So forget and forgo fragmentation of your psyche, dissemblance of your poise, and uncalled for exaggerated feelings of remorse and regret. You are not alone in sometimes falling short of goals. Don't become claustrophobic. Don't pen yourself in.

Cross train. This will not only help keep boredom at bay but will benefit your body by taxing muscles and motions in new ways, invigorating you physically and mentally. With a flexible manner you'll reach your goals faster than with the rigid and frigid form and formula.

Chapter 6

Walking, the perfect exercise, even for the eyes

If the desk jockeys at noon knew how the outdoors enthralls and captivates by smell, sight, and sound with its scenes of worry, wonder, and beauty, they will abide the drudgery of work with its relentless and picayune customs and habits, its unremitting monotony of the to-work-and-home commute, its same old same old lunch bag letdown, its unyielding demands for office conformity in playing politics and kissing ass—because they have risked the chance to see unique panoramas, vistas that send the observer from the humdrum and ho hum to the mountain pinnacles, stirring and swirling emotions of thankfulness, privilege and awe, as deep as the ocean and as wide as the prairie, and their place in the milieu will be rewarded by the streetscapes, that, every time experienced, calls for a reckoning that this day *yet again* proves that the midday stroll, saunter, or skip, with events unfolding unpredictable, delectable, formidable and unforgettable, sure as shooting beats Solitaire or Minesweeper at the old cubicle terminal.

A walk will do that for you.

On a beautiful sunny Friday in Toronto, I went for a noonday walk and, and, and—saw the monolith that is the Central Technical School, located at Bathurst and Harbord Street. The high school kids were cajoling and cavorting, hanging out, doing nothing particular with attitude, so far as I could see.

My eyes flashed to a young cop running with a pizza. I freaked as he ignored an unleashed Pit Bull. I freaked at the Pit Bull. I was taken aback by its owner, a Goth guy or girl possessed by an unprocessed blond mop of hair and a nonchalance bordering on insouciance about the dog and the cop. Then again, judging by the indeterminate appearance of the androgynous ambler, he she, or it, could have been simultaneously shuffling in a parallel world and not really there—here at all.

Flashback – near heart attack. High school sweethearts were lip locked. My jaw dropped. The smooch lasted for minutes. They'd gasp for air and go back at it. Everything's loosey goosey on a Friday. Oops, nearly fell of the curb. Now I'm peeking in a bistro. Oh, there is a second hand bookstore. "*Get With The Program!*" a book by Bob Greene, is front and center. Boy, I could use a lot of that. It is a #1 NY Times Best Seller! But at lunch I'm sold on walking. Got to go.

I was musing, gone, until disharmony banged and barged in. A 700-year-old man, give or take a century, wizened and perhaps wise beyond his years, was strumming and plucking the Chinese version of a sitar in cacophonous sequences and cadences. The noise was off putting but not nearly so upsetting as seeing the other listener who appeared out of nowhere (perhaps from another parallel world) beside me. He looked like an escaped convict, with his three pierced earrings in his schnozz, nastily underscored by chains draped all over his body. The chains reminded me of the ones Ebenezer Scrooge's old side kick, Jacob Marley, wore. And while this guy's complexion looked Marley-mortician-prepared casket ready, more than likely he was a genius computer geek whose balance sheet was better than mine. Now *that's* a crime.

I sped away, and up. Lunch hour, an extended hour to be sure, was near the end and I had to get to the St. Lawrence Market, on Front St. East, near Lower Jarvis. It foots Lake Ontario. There, I could buy chicken wings, nuclear size, about a foot wide if splayed apart. They taste great. I was immediately lost, imagining their savory flavor, drooling in anticipation, until I found my throat suddenly went dry. It cracked.

Why? It cracked because 20 yards away a skinny guy with droopy pants was baring his bare butt crack for all to bear. I turned to two ladies in passing whose gasps were the perfect audio for this visual rear spectacle and I said:

"Do we have to see this?" They giggled and nodded. The price you pay for walking. More free entertainment followed. Tugging and towing my double bagged eight chicken wings from the market I saw an unidentifiable object you can't put a price on. I turned to a policeman who was standing guard at a movie shoot and I blurted:

"Did you just see what I just saw?" He nodded and smiled. What we saw was a Unicar, an electric-powered, motorcycle-sized, V-shaped pilot project thing. Of course the policeman smiled; with the number of films shot in Toronto "Hollywood North" he has probably seen it all.

Indeed, anyone going for a walk at lunch in a big city or a small town can probably see it all, certainly enough to slake their visual thirst. And the added feature and definite benefit of these real life vignettes via voyage is that while you take in the pictures and events, with enough of these outings, say two to three per week, pretty soon you can take in that pant or skirt size too. Just goes to show you how fitting walking is.

Chapter 7
Working out and multitasking

What holds true for the work world holds true for fitness, namely that multitasking stinks as an effective practice. Way back…

"In 2006, University of California at Los Angeles researchers used MRI brain-mapping technology to determine that multitasking hurts one's ability to learn and remember information."

Mark Ellwood, a Toronto, Canada productivity expert and President of Pace Productivity Inc., "….wages a constant battle trying to persuade people that they can change how they spend their time and concentrate on one thing for unbroken stretches."

When you are weightlifting, focus on that repetition as though it was the only thing going. Beam in on what you hope to accomplish in your session and go about your business. Daydreaming is daft. Drop the muse, and focus, and you'll avoid falling over barbells some fool forgetfully left on the floor. Concentration means safety and superior results.

Chapter 8
Fitness and health role models

Children crave role models, seeking someone to learn from and look up to. Often we see these cute, innocent, inquisitive little faces peering at us and we think, yes, yes, I am making a difference. Then we have that sober second thought: children are built at low altitudes and look up to *everything*.

Seriously, should you, new to a fitness program, or a born-again health buff, need role models as guiding lights in your pursuits?

Depends. Having an example or a mentor to go by certainly can't hurt your cause, and thus there is nothing wrong with having the same, per se, but the real focus must be on you. Without you as the active person who watches what you eat and what you do, the role model is just window dressing, nothing more.

So if you want to do the job right, you have to do it yourself. Only you can take that bull by the horns and walk that walk, or lift that load.

Know what you will find? If you embark on this journey, even with the obligatory standard phobias, quirks, and fetishes we all have, and change from a pudgy to a more perfect physical paragon, you may have just become your very own personalized role model, and deservedly so.

Chapter 9
Training - rest and recuperation

On the one day out of seven, you take it easy, feel free to not read. Or at least not read the hectoring and sermonizing ads in newspapers, magazines, and flyers that besiege us to lose weight, gain muscle, go green, stop waste, reduce garbage, increase awareness, stand up, sit down, vote early, vote often, you get the idea.

Enough already.

On your day of rest, have your goal to contribute the square root of zero to the common weal.

There is absolutely nothing wrong with idly occupying space, fiddling around with nothing on one's plate, passing an eminently forgettable day, diligently unremarkable, unexplored, and unbecoming. This isn't tossing in the white towel; it's re-energizing one's batteries. Moreover, this seemingly uneventful day of inaction will balance out the win-at-all-costs, money-is-no-object, everything-goes, other six days of alpha hell.

Being dormant is not being down. Being a bystander is not being a passenger. Taking time to smell the roses is not an abdication of responsibility and an overindulgence in navel gazing. You've worked your tail off for six days. Put your feet up and let your hair down.

Chapter 10
Optimum workout times

What time of the day do you like to exercise or put it off? Are you an early bird or a night owl? Does the time of the day you do or don't work out impact on your general mental and physical well being? Jennifer Ackerman in a book titled *Sex Sleep Eat Drink Dream*, wrestles in depth with questions like these in her study of the body. In a nutshell, contrary to popular belief, it matters not a whit when you train.

Many of us do our best "stuff" at the crack of dawn. A lot of us, by necessity, go for a mid-day workout even though the health clubs are packed like sardines, with near night-club lineups for every exercising gizmo. And yet others, after tucking the kids into bed, find a late night exercise escape at the gym the perfect remedy to a stressful day.

Ackerman tells us there is not any scientific basis for the belief that early risers are richer, healthier, or happier. So enjoy your mid-day or evening workout, knowing you're not a scum-of-the-earth mud queen. Just get that exercise session in, no matter what the time.

When the mood hits, if the shoe fits and nothing is amiss, react and act because later you'll have time to reflect on the subject morning, noon, or night.

Chapter 11

Cardio or weights to start your workout?

Here is the answer to the chicken or the egg question of whether cardio or weights should start a workout.

This question has piqued the curiosity of many and the offered solution makes sense.

According to Alex Hutchinson who writes a "Jockology" column, it boils down to this: if you want to primarily benefit muscles begin with the weights, if you want to focus on cardio, begin with cardio. It's an either/or proposition.

The quotes below are taken from an excerpt of his book: "Which Comes First, Cardio or Weights?"

"Let's start with one incontrovertible fact: you can't fulfill your ultimate potential as both a weightlifter and a marathoner at the same time."

"This approach—starting with whichever activity is most important to you—is widely used by elite athletes."

"It turns out that the sequence of cellular events that leads to bigger muscles is determined in part by the same "master switch"—an enzyme called amp kinase—that controls adaptations for better endurance. But you can't have it both ways: the switch is set either to "bigger muscles" or to "better endurance," and the body can't instantly change from one setting to the other."

To strike a balance, alternate sessions beginning with cardio or weights. This will bode well.

Chapter 12

Exercise and beating back boredom

Eddie (not his real name) is 31 years old and getting bored. Not with the 31 years he has lived but with the three months of nightly pushups and sit ups he has diligently done. He is bored out of his brains and is looking to take it out on me, which makes sense given that it was my bright idea that got him on this track in the first place. And now with his new found strength and tone he could take me down a peg or two which aggravates me greatly given that I am only 5'4" dripping wet and if I were any shorter I'd be in a circus.

At any rate, he is feeling the monotony of an unchanging exercise routine. This hits most of us at one time or another. He asked me what I could suggest to relieve the monotony. Well one thing I certainly did not suggest was to throw in the towel and give up the program whole hog. For to stop or to quit is to surrender.

So I told him this. Think of the boredom as something that can certainly be downgraded with changes to his routines, in either time, function or both and if the blahs are not reduced to zero they are manageable at least, and if all else fails and he's still in a rut – nevertheless keep on that hamster wheel. Remember and rejoice in the compliments and smiles you get from friends and strangers at the new shape you have molded. These kudos, I stressed to Eddie, are the elixirs to counter ennui.

Chapter 13
Exercising—the hardest part

A trampoline teacher who principally makes his living as a children's fitness instructor confided to me about the hardest part of his own exercise program. He confessed the biggest hurdle was getting his feet out the door. I said, "huh?" and asked him what he meant and he replied:

"Just getting started," I cut in and said "come to think of it, that's a problem for me too," then I added "but you know what, every time, three minutes after, you are so glad you did. Right?"

He smiled and nodded, "Yup."

"But that initial effort," he grimaced, "is a tough bridge to cross."

To hear even this guy, fit as a fiddle at near 50, what with his trampoline and kids' fitness teaching, can also easily succumb to laziness, was an eye opener and jaw dropper. If this fellow will slack off and flounce around, just how many of us face this impediment in infinite?

So what's the solution? I asked him how he got off of his rump when the mood to laze was running rampant. He admitted that sloth-guilt would envelop him, and up he'd get. Perhaps the feeling guilty comes from religion. Possibly it doesn't. No matter. While recrimination isn't my bag, what whaps me over the head is but a simple truth, namely, *nothing bad* ever happened to me when I went on a walk or lifted some weights. That, then, is my prod to get started. Hopefully you will have, or will create, your own self-induced poker to get out there and shake a leg.

Chapter 14
Fitness injuries and recoveries

If the slightest hangnail hamstrings your fitness regimen, holding you on the sidelines for days on end, you have a low pain threshold. If you take a 90 mile per hour hardball in the face, wipe your jaw, shake your head, get back in the batter's box, ready for what may come your way, you have a high pain threshold. Most of us have average pain thresholds and before you think you might want to have a high pain threshold, think of Pedro.

Who is Pedro? Pedro was the horse my family owned growing up. It was half quarter horse-half thoroughbred and had a good disposition, as they say in the industry. It also had absolutely no feelings in its lower front legs. The nerves had been destroyed, I can't remember the circumstances, and I recall telling my dad that must be great for Pedro and he said, no, not really, as its legs could be on fire and he would not feel a thing. Awareness of pain is needed. Insulation from pain is detrimental.

And so it goes with an injury from sport or exercise. You *must* listen to your body and hear what it tells you. If it screams in pain you are in trouble, if the scream is a low throb maybe you are overtraining; if you feel muscle stiffness, not soreness, chances are no real harm has been done and all systems are go, after a couple of days of rest.

But what should you do when actual injury does occur? What are the steps to heal, and then recover? We've all read about elite athletes coming back from injuries too soon. They aggravate the injury. And then boom, they are out of action.

(Or there are special so-lame cases like that of Chicago Cubs baseball slugger Sammy Sosa who was put on the disabled list for back injuries because of *sneezing*.)

Speaking of games...

I heard something this morning that surprised me, but upon reflection made eminent sense. A bunch of gents were talking of outdoor activities what with spring now here. One piped up:

"Do you know which sport has the most injuries?"

Everybody passed and he answered, "Softball."

Face it, most us are recreational players and head out to play a few innings woefully unprepared in ligament, tendon, and muscle flexibility and strength. Pulled muscles and torn groins go hand in hand with huffing and puffing while chugging along the base paths culminating with the slide into base. Yeah, you're safe but you are out of the game in awful pain. And who is to blame? An ounce of prevention is worth a pound of cure. Warm up before any game, don't overdo it, and don't go for the gusto and glory if out of shape generally, or out of game shape specifically.

With professional athletes, under pressure from management and fans to perform (and to not sneeze or cough) this happens more often than with the amateur athlete in a sport nobody, save for the athlete and maybe their mother, cares anything about. Expectations are astronomically higher for the former.

But to you, amateur, pro, or tweener, the possibility of injury could be a potential screw-up on your path to success.

I was glancing through my daily paper's health section and learned what a certain Dr. Tim Rindlisbacher says:

"The most confident prediction we can make is that if you stay focused, take it slow and set reasonable goals, you can come back from a minor injury quickly, and from a major injury in time."

I'm sure we will all be focused on our injury and its aftermath, but I'm also sure that the taking of things too quickly at a new regimen's outset and setting unreasonable, outlandish goals is where most of us fall down on the job. We're setting ourselves up for failure from the get go.

In the final analysis Dr. Rindlisbacher offers common sense and perspective:

"So don't measure your own injuries and recovery by professional sports standards. Take it all with a chunk of salt and find a more positive strategy for coping with your injury and working at recovery."

Not sure where one should find a more positive strategy. Under the couch? Keep the faith, and find your moxy and mettle within, I suppose, is what the doctor means - that - and maintaining in training paramount principles of proper form and moderation, and those principles, coupled with a prayer or two, will probably prevent injury in the first place.

Method Two: The personal trainer route

Chapter 15
Why method two? The big sleep

Between Method One and Method Two, I went into a long sleep (16 months or so). Actually that is not quite true, it might have been 17 months.

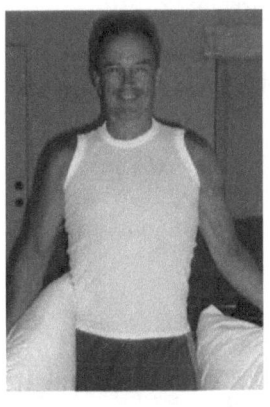 The background is that I was forced to hibernate from my job when I, along with a hundred others, were right sized, downsized, ostracized, and atomized right out of work. So I plopped myself down in front of my computer, armed with cigarettes, booze, ice cream, chocolate sauce, pistachio nuts and whatever else was bad for me within arm's reach—and the weight I had lost following Method One, and kept off until late 2008, came back faster than a boomerang on bennies, whilst I taught myself the basics of video making and writing-blogging. The jury's out on whether I pass muster with video making and writing-blogging but anyone who saw me could easily render a decision on my physical condition: during the 16 months my weight shot up again to 205 pounds.

Me, settling in for my big sleep of 16 months...

Once I woke up I decided to prove to myself, and to you dear reader, that hiring a personal trainer could be the best thing going to lose fat and get fit.

Chapter 16

What happens if you employ a personal fitness trainer?

These three pictures show how quickly true change can occur when one enlists the help of a professional—and wisely follows that person's advice—to the letter.

Weight starting point – 205 pounds (92 kilograms) November 2, 2010.

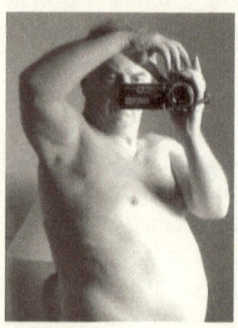

Looks like I'm carrying twins, huh? I was certainly carrying a lot of angst and self-loathing. Shot before my first session with my fitness trainer.

Weight and shape after 26 sessions: 168 pounds (76 kilograms) on January 12, 2011. The 27th was a tutorial prep primer for continuing my conditioning without a trainer.

After 26 sessions with the fitness trainer, plus walking on my own slightly over 10 miles (16.09 kilometers) per day, I dropped an average .51 pounds (233.15 grams) daily. Or a total of 37 pounds (16 kilograms) from Nov. 2nd, 2010 to Jan. 12th, 2011. The calories lost per day equaled about 1,799.

Here is what happened when I decided to follow through on my own: – 144 pounds (65 kilograms) – April 13, 2011.

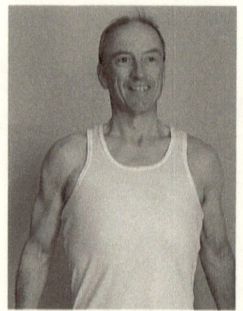

Probably a bit too "Skinny Minnie" for some, but after being a balloon, it's hard not to push the envelope in the other direction... For better or for worse: 144 pounds as at April 13, 2011

For those that want the straight goods, the scoop, the "skinny"—here in a nutshell was what I did, and did not do, using Method Two with the personal fitness trainer.

Method	2
Smoking	N
Alcohol	N
Junk food	N
Walking	Y
Elliptical	Y
Weight training	Y
Tracking progress	Y
Weigh ins – scale	Y
Fitness trainer	Y
Pounds lost	37*
Time taken	72 days
Average pounds lost per day	0.514
Average grams lost per day	233.15

*For method 2 the total lost was 61 pounds (27 kg), in just under 6 months (173 days), with the last 24 pounds coming off after my session with my trainer ended.

The average pounds, therefore, lost per day with method 2 before and after my fitness trainer was 61 pounds/173 days = 0.353 lost per day (grams 160.12 per day)

The table above, while clean and pristine, doesn't begin to tell the harrowing tale of strenuous exertion that unfolded, and that was just in the introductory interview with my prospective fitness trainer. When I heard I had to cut milk from my diet, I darn near went fetal. When I was told that cigarettes and booze also had to be given the big heave-ho, I damn near turtled, cursing and cussing, simpering like a wimp.

On the other hand, consider: I was paying some pretty large bucks for the 27 sessions, try $1,800 dollars, and I vowed to listen, learn and obey every suggestion, order, command, and fiat that emanated from my personal Hitler health harridan. Otherwise what would be the point?

The larger question was, what if we didn't click? We've all had teachers we admired and that could inspire and we've all had teachers that should perspire because they stunk as instructors. My initial impression of my trainer was good.

But, back to the changes I vowed to make immediately after our chat before session number one. I was sorry to see milk go, and was near hyperventilating at the thought of no junk food crossing my lips for the next nine weeks (three sessions per week) but my instructor stressed, and this jolted me, that dietary choices accounted for 70% of the success one would have in their quest to lose weight. I glommed on that fact harder than an NRA member might hug a shotgun, and arbitrarily decided that foregoing chips, ice cream, popcorn, butter, bread and whatnot would be more than half the battle.

Ok, easy peasy stuff there, but what about quitting drinking and smoking? I had tried about eight times previously to quit smoking and largely had been spectacularly unsuccessful, with one nine-week abstinence my longest period without butts on record. Every time I had tried to quit smoking I had kept on drinking rum and cokes, and black Russians, and beers and I'd light up after the first drink, or the first swig because I think, at least for me, that the laws of physics and societal malarkey made it immutable and non-debatable that booze and cigarettes must blend and bond and be taken together. So on this 9th attempt I got smart and cut out the booze too. (So far, so good. I have not tasted or inhaled either for two years plus. Only in the spring of 2013 have I had a couple of beers here and there with no cigarettes. But at the first sign of cravings for the demon weed, I'll stop having a social drink or two again.)

In a way it was easier to quit both habits cold turkey, and ban the junk food at the same time, and change the portions of my meals and the composition of same, while taking these three killer weight sessions per week. When I freaked out during quiet times, I never could pin down exactly which trigger was pissing me off and making it difficult for me to make a decision.

How best to gripe? Should I make acquaintances I will certainly later want to lose and complain interminably to them, thereby having them cast me off later as a chronic egocentric bore? Should I push "the buttons" of a significant other while we are in the down slope of a relationship, and set them off with incessant carping? Or should I act my age, as a mature middle-aged man well past 50, and do what comes naturally, that is, rattle and babble to myself out loud?

I chose the latter. But blabbing out loud in a gym could be a life ending move, some Hercules or Amazon could throw a weight my way. So I decided that walking would be the avenue, the path, the road, the route I'd take with arguing with myself over all my abstinence and alteration adaptations. Thus, from Nov. 2nd 2010 to Jan 12th 2011, I walked like a crazy old coot, averaging *over 10 miles (16.09 kilometers) daily.*

Apart from the question as to how in their right mind anyone with a life worth living has time to traipse for 10+ miles per day, where on God's green earth could such be done without being whapped by the vagaries and vicissitudes of rain, snow, sleet, smog, "stuff" you know?

Got to tell you, I was in a fog about that one. And then it hit me. I'd get my personal trainer and my walking tied together and kick my bunch of lousy life habits and raise a new fit, fine me in a little nook of nirvana, more commonly known on this planet earth as Palm Springs, California. Here are three airport terminal shots that should persuade you. Tweet and Twitter.

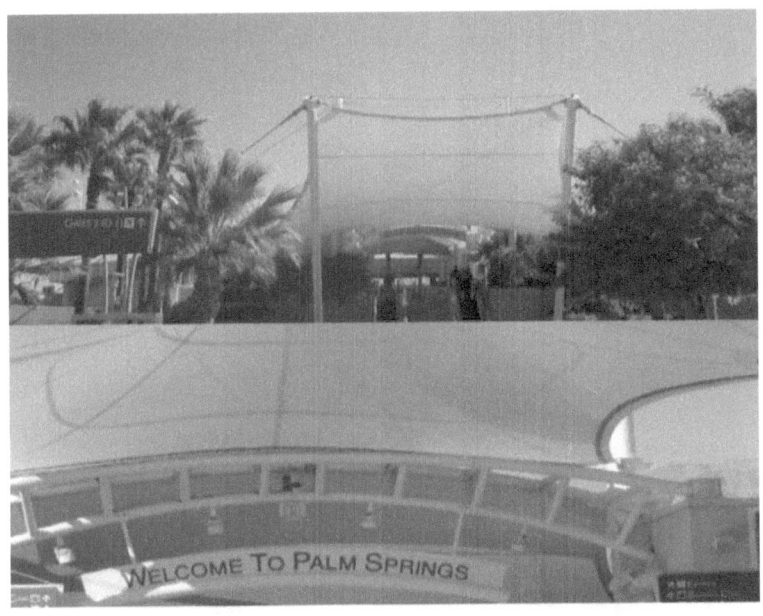

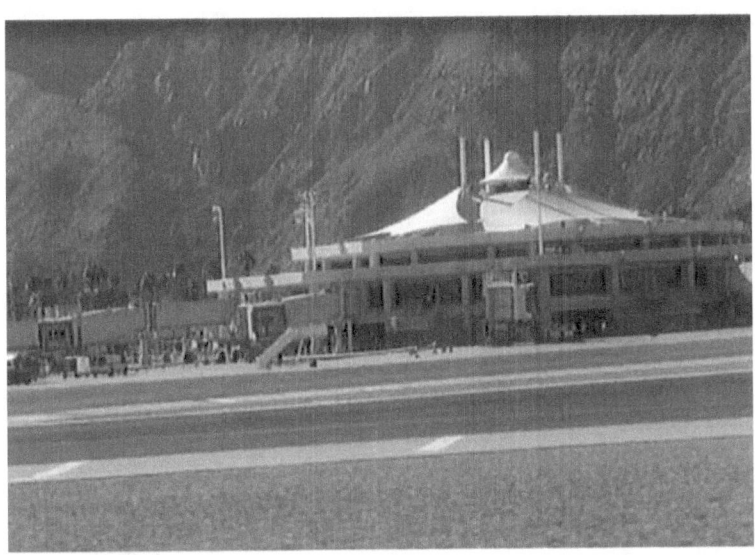

Chapter 17
So let's see what a Palm Springs fitness instructor can do. . .

Palm Springs in sizzling, sunny, Southern California is a state of mind, a desert-des-
sert, a slice of perfection pie sitting atop a fault line, the San Andreas Fault, which
is more garishly threatening to live through and view than your usual Hollywood
starlet botched-up face job. The fabulously rich and jet-lagged jaded have made
their homes here, and now, thanks to the U.S. real estate marketing cratering faster
than a Florida sinkhole, so can you.

(Of course, some residences have held their value. For $50 million big ones you
can pick up Bob Hope's estate.)

And Palm Desert, just southeast from Palm Springs, is even better. And that,
specifically, was where I'd do my walking and get my fitness sessions in with my
personal trainer. But first you land at the sharpest, snazziest, coolest—even on a
scorching day—airport, the out-of-this-world Palm Springs International Airport,
and the scent of flora, bathed in dry desert air and the sight of the craggy mountains
that caress the airport, seemingly scoots the nauseas fumes of aviation fuel into
some kind of netherworld.

And the weather, for you data hounds, can only be technically described as first
rate. When my flight landed around 2 in the afternoon, weather was performing to
form. The weather is conveniently perfect with average temperatures cruising in at
73.9 degrees Fahrenheit, with yearly precipitation inching in at 5.2, enough to make
it interesting.

What is even more interesting is how just *leaving* Palm Springs is a heavenly
dream, if you are more depressed than hell. Most airports these days are cattle runs,
where the hoi-polloi of all hues queue with expressions ranging from purple rage
to pallid resignation. Not this puppy. The lineups, and this is surprising, given the
popularity of this vacation Valhalla, seem smaller. And classier. There are no white
trash boogers, or buggers or horkers or hobos here. Even if you get felt up, it feels
more like a high-priced hooker or gigolo are doing the dirty pat-down, as opposed
to an underpaid Transport Security Administration (TSA) employee. Their uni-
forms look somewhat clean. They don't have signs that say "I got no crabs, no lice,

no vermin of any variety to speak of, at least today." Sometimes they smile. I read that somewhere.

Boy, sorry, got way off track.

First, I had to put up with the typical U.S. airport situation in 2010. Right after the foreplay of having your organs set a-flutter and afire by a complete stranger with X-ray attendants acting as voyeurs and bin passer backers playing peeping Toms, your escape from reality continues, owing to the aforementioned crummy, crappy US economy. The prices you pay for a hackneyed, dried out airport tuna sandwich with limp lettuce aren't egregiously gouge-like: you don't have to take out a second mortgage for it.

But people tell you, just by looking at them, there's a lot of financing finagling and funding footwork going on to change those proverbial feet of clay into something delightful and demure. Or at least that's the intent of the money machinations. If you can get past the facial abominations, the bean bag breasts, the paper mache posteriors, the lopsided lips, the cement cheekbones, the nipped noses, the rebar sashaying hips - and all these evident on the cougar airline stewardesses - you gotta see the passengers and locals - you'll find Palm Springs real, almost down-home like.

And it was to be my home in November 2007 for part of Method One, and again in 2010 for Method Two, with the fitness trainer.

That was a reason I had misgivings and apprehensions about the fitness trainer gambit. Yet, by Jove, I realized the construction in these parts is a treasure trove of rehabilitation, renovation and resurrection. Just think what an experienced fitness pro could do. They'd do a complete teardown of my execrable edifice, stage a nexus neighborhood in transition phase, and finish off in a rebuild, created to-last-for-all-seasons, gild.

Then I'd take a stroll down El Paseo a glitzy, ritzy super-high-end retail shopping district and contrast architectural grace with the shopping face: often a face mis

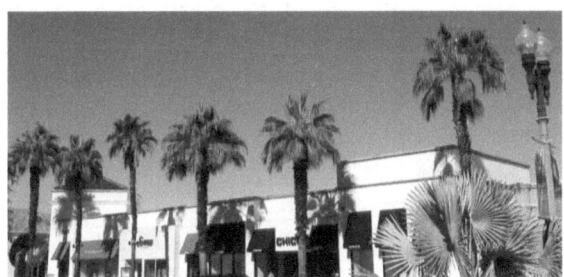

placed, a face needing mace, a face with no taste... and I'd wonder if the personal fitness coach was the way to go... Then I'd do a 180 turn. Heck, if women can be made virgins again, perhaps my form could return to its firm foundations. In Palm Springs, anything is possible and nothing is improbable on the makeover menu. The old abdominoplasty (Tummy Tuck) is an entree crowd favorite. Down here taking short cuts (pun intended) to success is practically mandatory. A sense of calm would wash over me. Then a chill of consternation, as I'd read that the only thing shaking larger than the earthquakes here are the tremors and tirades from testy husbands and ticked-off wives who are asked for their opinions on their mates' latest, not so greatest, surgery jobs.

What about Job One, me?

I wasn't sure if I wanted someone who empathized with my roly-poly shape or someone emphatic to change it. Would a tough taskmaster, ready to break and bend my body by sheer force of iron will, be best? In short, did I want a "players" coach or a "coaches" coach?

I took a cab to a city just a bit south and east of Palm Desert, La Quinta. That's where a relative had arranged an appointment to interview with a fitness trainer he had used—and raved about. At 11 AM, while talking to the administrator, something out of left field, or at least to my left, caught my eye.

Oh, my. I saw a great mop of red hair atop an awesome body. He, this Hercules, must have had ESP. He saw me and got into a football three-point stance. He was going to flatten me.

It worked. I was, so to speak, bowled over, and grateful he spared me physically. I was also now putty in his hands. I was a supplicant to whatever would come my way, so long as it came from him. I was bonded to this guy. It took all of ten seconds. And we hadn't even exchanged hellos.

When I said I was thinking of getting a fitness trainer once I was in a bit better shape, he flatly contradicted me and said I had to man up and hire one right away. I nodded instantly. When I ventured that half hour sessions would be best he stopped me cold and said hour ones were the way to go. I nodded meekly. When I said I thought 15 sessions ought to do the trick he said, nope, I was looking at 27 sessions, minimum. I said yup, nodding slavishly. When I said I'd like a female trainer—he didn't argue with that—and I felt so strong, so powerful, so potent, so omnipotent, I didn't even nod.

I was too busy kissing his feet.

But it was to be my feet that would, along with my fitness sessions, see me through from fat guy to fit guy in Method Two.

And for those sessions that were particularly arduous and awful, for therapy, I managed to scribble down what the heck was happening to my psyche and physique. Which follows.

Session 1 Nov. 15th 2010

Oh, isn't everything fun on the first full day of anything! Even Day One of school bordered on enjoyable some years, as I remember, and in a sense this was like class. Boy, are there a lot of new machines I can—and will—be using, from what I gather. And little did I know that my grunting, giving it my all for four sets of 20 each on them, on this, and on that again, was not unlike a woman in childbirth without an epidural. The difference is, when I got home after labor I delivered rants not rug rats.

Nov. 16th 2010. My trainer warned me that, quite often, muscle stiffness occurs 36 hours after serious exertion, not 24 hours. Quite right. Almost to the hour, in my case. It is not a debilitating stiffness but it did help me realize that I must walk on my off days and listen to my body. I can tell that I'll be working harder with my trainer than I would ever do on my own. I sure don't miss alcohol and cigarettes so far, given that every muscle group is twinging and tweaking. It's like I've got a new family visiting and I don't have time to think about how I'm hard done by, and put out by, what I'm missing. What good would a bottle of booze do anyway when I'm too stiff and spent to reach into the cupboard to get it?

Session 2 Nov. 17th 2010

An absolute, hour long, killer. I normally never sweat while working with weights or machines. But this workout was abnormal. It's good to know my ticker can tock like crazy. (The last time I felt my heart beat this fast and hard was every time I ask a girl to dance.)

I threatened to quit—sort of joking. Then I resorted to offering bribes so my trainer would cut back. But my trainer was already onto my game. She doesn't let me cheat, too often, by running away from her for water from the fountain. I tested her, seeing if I could take a water break every five minutes, but she said no way. And for this I pay? And she knows exactly how to space out an hour, keeping the exercises different and my emotions apparent and running at a fever pitch. Great workout. My best hour ever.

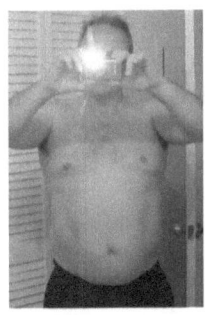

Nov. 17th 2010. After Session 2. I forgot to weigh myself. Too tired. I could barely lift this tiny camera.

Session 3 Nov. 19th 2010

This is all I remember saying to my trainer: "Every part that is stiff on me I owe to you." Geez, as soon as I said it, I realized that didn't sound good, if said to a female employee. But we both had a good laugh. Enough said.

Session 4 Nov. 22nd 2010

No commentary for this session other than to note that the picture below, taken before the session, shows a four pound drop from 205 to 201 pounds.

I dropped four pounds to now weigh 201 pounds as at Nov. 22nd.

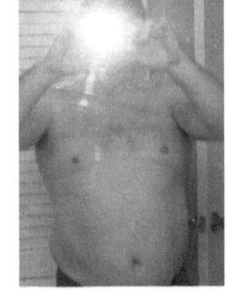

Session 5 Nov. 24th 2010

But nothing in life is easy. The never-ending hour never seems to end. I thought my triceps would wilt doing dips and then my torturer set and freed the chin up machine to run roughshod over me. Luckily she picked up on my quivers and shakes and set the weight at 50% of my body weight.

I was ready to buy her a diamond right then and there.

But then I had to do a million repetitions and my mood of glee turned to a mood of grumpy, with grins to grimaces, and I remembered diamond is made of carbon... the best I could come up with was to try and exhale carbon dioxide in her direction.

She shucked that off and she's certainly a professional in shushing off my complaining and caterwauling. In spite of myself, I think I'm getting quite a bit stronger and the fact that she assigns clearly defined repetitions and sets is critical to my improvement. Without her targets and her encouragement, I'm sure I'd slack off and do less. This is why I'm paying the big bucks. It could be the best money I've ever spent.

Session 6 Nov. 27th 2010

Fortunately this session, while good verging on great, was held not on Friday, but on Saturday, which allowed the 36 hour-later stiff period from Wednesday's workout to subside. So I was just fine on Saturday. I only felt lingering stiffness when I sat, stood, sauntered and spoke. Truthfully, since session one I have been tender all over. My trainer did the Turkey Trot Thanksgiving run on Thursday and averaged about 8 minutes per mile. The race started at 7am and it is cold in the Coachella Valley then at this time of year. She asked me if I wanted to go. I said no. Like the millions of turkeys to be devoured on Thanksgiving, I had been boiled, baked, and fried on Wednesday, all at once.

Session 7 Nov. 29th 2010

I love the club when I leave it and I like trying to get my instructor off her game when I'm at it. Why do I do this? To get out of doing so many exercises, or at least to space out the repetitions. And how do I do this? By asking her every question under the sun before I get on to a new machine, or between sets. I ask her of family, of friends, of near friends, of acquaintances, of strangers, of enemies, of celebrities, of people she met once, of people she'd like to meet, of people that are nearly dead, of people that have long since bit the dust, anything to avoid the workout.

Session 9 Dec. 3rd 2010

No commentary, but this picture tells a tale of progress, even if that progress seems, visually, almost unnoticeable. Still, the scale doesn't lie.

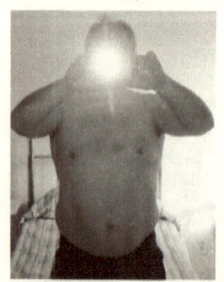

From Nov. 2nd to Dec. 3rd after nine sessions, I now weigh 198 pounds. Total weight loss so far - seven pounds.

Session 12 Dec. 10th 2010

I am so tired I'm delirious. I certainly feel like I'm a special needs client and all I really need, especially now, is to stop exercising my obliques on this infernal machine. I'm trying to fake out my instructor, show her how deluded I've become by calling her Patty, Janet, Margo— none of which she answers to, none being her actual name.

Cripes. Susan has just ordered me to do another set. Damn you, Louise.

Session 13 Dec. 13th 2010

Today, Dec. 13, my body fat rolled in at 32.8%. (My trainer uses a dastardly contraption to calculate same.) That was neither fish nor fowl but what followed shortly afterwards was fishy. I had to try to climb on top of the "Everest" sit-up bench at a slant so steep the blood immediately rushed to my feet—and that was even before I clambered on to the thing. (My body was getting prepared because in a few seconds the blood would reverse flow and rush immediately to my head once propped onto the board.)

And once I was basically in a headstand position my instructor passed me a two pound ball and told me to do a sit up and pass the ball back to her. She had to be kidding. But this was no joke. I failed, failed miserably, for ten repetitions worth and those alone, coupled with my burning shame, frustration, and embarrassment had to move the body fat measurement down big time, for next time.

Or so I hoped…

Session 15 Dec. 17th 2010

This was the first session where total focus was on particular body parts. Throughout the first 14 sessions we both agreed my body would not be able to withstand beaming in on certain sectors. Or look at it this way: All parts needed to be worked on slowly and surely so that progress would be made everywhere. But today she basically said we had to move from Grade One to Grade Two and that the chest, shoulders, and back would be the bearers of bulk loading with abs, as always, at the end. It's a heckuva way to end a workout, crunching and keeled over in pain. But I wouldn't have it any other way. Let me put that another way. She wouldn't.

Session 16 Dec. 20th 2010

Normally when you're a guy for example, and a member of the opposite sex says, "You can see it going down," it would be cause for alarm, if not a cause for a complete and utter mental breakdown. And a dash to the drugstore. But in this case the significant other was my personal fitness trainer and she was, I think, referring to my weight.

Indeed before this 16th session, in which we did the measurement weigh in and body fat totals, she asked, "Where are you?" after my body fat came in at 31%, a drop of 1.8% from Dec. 13. This was my cue to tell her of a similar comment I heard the first time I lost weight (about 50 pounds at that specific time, while using Method 1). An old friend saw me in the elevator and said "Where did you go?" Well, I am still here, more aware, acute, and alive than ever, but nevertheless 40 to 50 pounds above where I want to be. When my instructor gave me the high five for good numbers, I thought that might buy me out of my 16th session but, alas, that *so* did not happen.

Session 18 Dec. 24th 2010

Boy, was I in the Christmas spirit this 24th of December. With a twist. Like a child who hides behind the rocking chair in the hopes of seeing Santa Claus, I hid too. Behind Nautilus machines so my Grinch trainer wouldn't see me. But I'm still roly-poly so I stood out. And then I gave all I had carrying out the exercises she had diabolically presented me.

But she has truly given me a great gift. This Christmas season I won't be eating all the cookies, sweets, and other goodies that abound. Though I've certainly got the stomach for them, I don't have the cravings. In any event, my trainer had given me a list of acceptable or recommended foods. So I won't have to drop an extra ten pounds or so of holiday heft. My fitness program can continue uninterrupted.

Session 19 Dec. 27th 2010

No verbiage today, and no picture either, but this chart showing my weight loss and body fat reductions provides a snapshot of the progress. Nov. 29th I weighed 201 pounds with 36.3% body fat. Dec. 27th I was at 180 and 31% respectively.

Session 20 Dec. 29th 2010

I now have a new strategy for bribery! From now on, whenever I'm training I'm going to be liquid, and that's over and above my plethora of water breaks. Yeah, I'm going to be flush with cash. And not to bribe my trainer to stop doing what I'm paying her to do, but to slip other slippery exercisers bills to take machines just before I'm set to get on them, thus throwing a monkey wrench into the whole shebang. I'll frustrate my fitness schedule completely. Works for me. Even if it is against everything I'm ostensibly here to do. Aren't us spineless folks supposed to be conflicted? This is war! And being at war with myself, I'm the first casualty.

New Year's Resolution Dec. 31st 2010

Well I can thank my personal trainer for one thing. Several things, in fact. Since starting in with this routine Nov. 15th I have quit smoking, stopped drinking, overhauled my diet choices, and hacked my meal portions. Therefore my New Year's resolution and wish is but this: to keep on keeping on with the same. Steady as she goes, Skipper.

Session 22 Jan. 3rd 2011

It is the look of disgust that gets to you first. The sneer, the disdain, and the utter revilement and derision that one's fitness trainer shows when one (me) collapses on the slanted sit up board. But I deserved the brickbat. I was pretty useless today. I couldn't even get my feet properly locked in up top without her help. After that it was all downhill. In all ways.

Session 24 Jan. 7th 2011

Is it possible that rolling a ball up a wall could be so much fun? On the face of it, the task does not appear that difficult, except that the ball weighs an anchor's worth and except that I am punched after too many squats and too many lunges, so by the time the malevolently grinning trainer demands this deed, I am finito. And it's barely noon.

Session 26 Jan. 12th 2011

As it turned out my last workout session was 26. (The 27th session was intended for photos of equipment and tips to remember going forward upon my return home.) My trainer did lead me through all the machines my next club stop in Calgary might have. And we reviewed basics—never let the knee go in front of the toes on a lunge, make sure the knees are parallel with the hinges on a hamstring or quadriceps machine, etc. And I wasn't to forget to do sit ups on the slanted board and I was not to cheat on the counting. And I was to keep her posted and maintain my new dietary choices.

And, though we didn't discuss it, I was determined to not start drinking or smoking again. The final picture after Session 26, with the total weight loss data, is at the front of this chapter. Basically I lost 37 pounds from Nov. 2nd 2010 to Jan. 12th 2011. My trainer was the brunt of good-spirited barbs but I owe her a huge thank you for changing my diet and freeing me up from my impediments and detriments of smoking and drinking. In actual fact Adrienna Collins was my personal trainer. She worked me over at World Gym in Palm Desert. Thanks so much Adrienna, you are the best!

Now, a word about fitness trainers: Before hiring one, my opinion on the profession was at best—neutral, at worst—uninformed. Let's take a look back to the relatively early days (15 to 20 years ago) of how trainers came to be a part of personal fitness.

Chapter 18
The merits of personal fitness trainers

Do you remember the good old days and decades when caring club staff roamed our gym clubs, handing out free fitness advice? I found one gentleman at my old health club very helpful. He saved me *thousands of instances* of unnecessary pain. All it cost me was to shut up for a few minutes and listen to what he had to say.

I had been a member for about 10 years. It was an early Saturday morning, I think, and hardly anyone else was around. It took me a while but I summoned up the nerve to tell him my problem. I should not have been so nervous. He and others I spoke to later would stop in their tracks when I tossed a question their way, perk up, and explain the equipment, routines, methods, and best practices. On the ball. And available. They were an unrecognized asset for most. But in my time there I only had this one question, prefaced by a barely decipherable description.

"My right big toenail is purple and you won't, it's you know, this… it's kinda like I have two toe nails, I can't cut them, I have to wait until they are way over the toe—it's gross—and I stub it 'cause it's way out there and… have you heard of this?"

"Are you a runner?"

"Yeah, lately I've been putting on the miles."

"How many per week?"

"I don't know maybe 20, a couple of times 30, who knows?"

"Where do you run?"

"Here, Toronto."

"No, no I mean do you run at a track, grass—?"

"The track at my high school sometimes, but mostly, you know, around home, sidewalks."

"No more sidewalks."

"What? I'd think, you know, they're safer—no cars, accidents. What's wrong?"

"Concrete is harder than pavement."

"I didn't know that."

"Yeah and with your mileage—do you run heel to toe or mostly on the balls of your feet?"

"I'm a clomper, I tried the heel to toe but my shins—one of those up and down guys, tendons, I don't know, would start with the dull pain, so I'm guess I'm basically a clomper."

"You should see a doctor about that."

"What's a doctor going to do?"

"Well you're hitting—any time you whack something against a hard… you are looking at … say your right nail it's hitting the ground 7,000 times per day."

"No, no, no."

"Oh sure, 'cause don't forget you are walking too, that all counts."

Being a man, I did not see a doctor. But I was bright enough to see his reasoning regarding what type of surfaces I should, and should not, run on and I was smarter still to put his advice to use from that day forward.

As it turned out, I lost that nail. It was pretty much a dead duck but I did gain insight: some pain, to the hurtful tune of 7,000 steps or strides per day damaging shins, tendons and the like, is not inflicted by voodoo, or bad luck, or dreadful circumstances, or by fluke, but by one's own carelessness and/or lack of awareness. They say you get what you pay for, on the premise that anything free is going to be worthless or even harmful, but there are exceptions to such bromides and this one is a good example.

And yes, over time, gym attendants have changed roles from when they staffed clubs in the 1980's and 1990's. They are still in our gyms and health clubs but have, in this new millennium, morphed into fee-based, advice-by-the-adjective, vouchsafed-by-the-verb, personal trainers. Oh, personal trainers will pick up a barbell for you, or move weights out of the way, if you are their client. For the hour. Otherwise, it is every step for itself. And be careful out there; it is a phys-ed jungle.

Nowadays, if one is out of sorts (as most of us are), and has a burning question, and can't wait to blurt it out, does one dare to do so? Today's personal trainers are impressive physical specimens to a man and a woman. They impress. They give one the impression that if a question were asked, even "Where is the washroom?" one would be up on harassment charges like that, lickety split, no seconds flat.

There is, of course, the money issue. Take a minute to think about whether you can brave their fees, fees that range anywhere from $40 to $60 for a half an hour and $80 upwards to $180 plus for an hour. You are guaranteed to lose weight. You'd be too scared not to. And even if you weren't, those fees would scare one svelte.

All that said, for many, these personal trainers are the best thing to hit the industry, next to the steam room. They have, individually and as a group, honed, buffed and primped and pushed us farther than we wished to go physically and athletically. Every time we see one, we get right with the program and train ourselves, immediately.

Okay, on to Method Three.

Chapter 19

Why method three? To test the fantastic five diet for rapid weight loss, huge $savings, and fitness personal bests

Method Three: The Controlled Diet Route

There is nothing wrong with someone weighing 191.4 pounds (86 kilograms) on a Thursday February 2, 2012—nothing wrong with it, but certainly nothing right with it—given that this is the *third time* my weight has soared to the heavy heights of near, or over, 200 pounds. And there is *definitely* nothing wrong with weighing a relatively scant 160.6 pounds (72 kilograms) less than two months later…

Now, I should make clear that I did *not* fall off the wagon. I let myself gain the weight deliberately. It was a controlled experiment. I wanted to see what would happen if I focused systematically on a controlled diet instead of on fitness, as in Method Two. I did, however, maintain a fitness routine and recorded the results, as they related to diet change.

More generally, I wanted to demonstrate something beyond the porcine round-ness on display in the first photo below: *The same person can use different methods successfully to drop fat, lose weight, add muscle, and gain shape.* Watch what happened this time around.

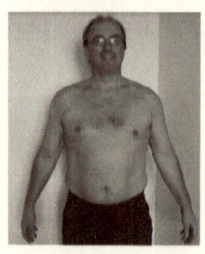

But zounds, gaining weight was a breeze! From August 2011 to the beginning of February, I went on a rip-roaring tear—eating, feasting, forking, shoveling and smashing junk food down my pie hole, morning, mid-morning, noon, mid-afternoon, dusk, evening, and night.

86 kg 191.4 lbs 2 Feb. 2012

But by February 1st 2012, all I had proven was that I was wide. I crushed the scale at 197 pounds.

Why didn't I take a picture at 197 pounds? Because I wasn't sure how the first day with my new food choices and regular exercise routine would pan out. But since it did so splendidly, I whipped out my camera and searched for a room big enough to fit my frame in—and here I am at 191.4 pounds.

So the picture captures the second day on my new "fit-to-be-tied, fly-right, get-on-the-straight-and-narrow, and-smarten-up-while-you're-at-it" foray into diet. I had dropped 5.6 pounds overnight.

72 kg 160.6 lbs 21 March 2012

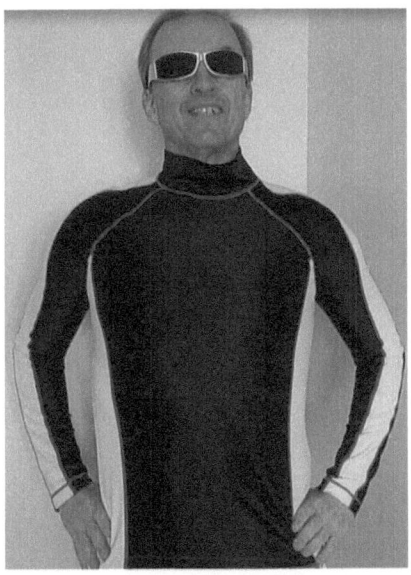

And the big drop was due to 5.25 miles (8.45 kilometers) walking, a weights workout, and a big chuck.

The big chuck: I poured the homogenized milk down the sink, threw out the chicken wings, put the George Foreman cooker in dry docks, gave away the Jalapeño chips, and put two tall glasses of water in the fridge. I then bought four bags of green split pea legumes (a buck each), a bag of spinach (can be eaten raw or cooked), two dozen eggs, seven red grapefruit (for the fat-burning molecules), and a bag of Spanish or Sweet onions. (The latter look almost exactly the same.) I called these foods my Fantastic Five.

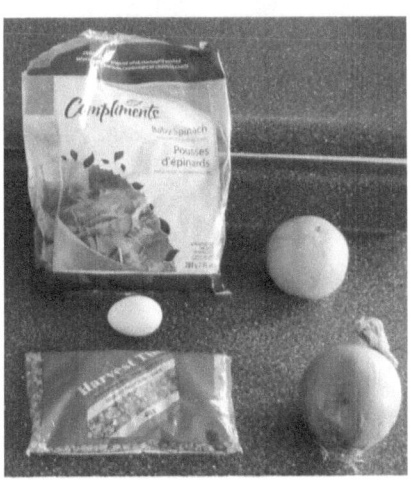

Using them, I was going to lose the weight I had deliberately put on and become a new man, or a lean man anyway.

Why did I choose these foods? I had used them, in some instances, though not regularly, in Method Two. I liked the taste of all of them. I knew them to be low in the caloric "addition to the body" factor. They are readily available in most supermarkets. They are very easy to cook with. And being quite inexpensive, I knew they'd be perfect to prove that losing fat, and gaining fitness, can be done on a limited budget.

45

Method Three, in retrospect, was, I must emphasize this again, super easy on the pocketbook and just as easy in the kitchen. And the pounds melted off easily too. In fact, it was so easy as to be a bit of a ho-hum, hum-drum affair. To be truthful here, after a couple of weeks on just five food choices, the lack of diversity in comestibles' taste, type, and texture did wear a bit thin. But I was wearing *a lot* thinner, too, daily. And this inexorable, near inevitable progress, dulled any pangs of regret over a fairly pedestrian menu.

Here's what I did, and did not do, with Method Three.

Method	3
Smoking	N
Alcohol	N
Junk food	N
Walking	Y
Elliptical	Y
Weight training	Y
Tracking progress	Y
Weigh ins – scale	Y
Fitness trainer	N
Pounds lost	36
Time taken	50 days
Average pounds lost per day	0.72
Average grams lost per day	326.59

Let's look at the chart and pictures below. Then I'll detail how easy Method Three was on all accounts and how it could, in whole or in part, work for you.

Starting weight: 197 pounds (89 kg). Total pounds lost = 36.4 (kg 16).

Ending weight: 160.6 pounds (72 kg). Lost daily average = .72 of a pound (327 grams.)

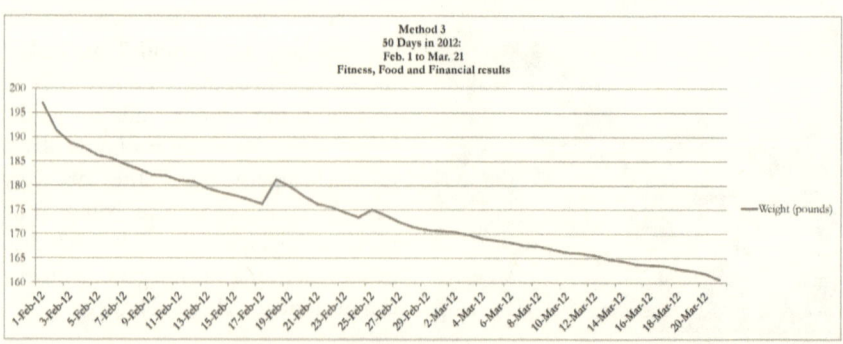

Method 3
50 Days in 2012:
Feb. 1 to Mar. 21
Fitness, Food and Financial results

Fat, food, and financial facts

50 days: Lost weight in 48 of them. The two upward blips were for a buffet one night and for a heaping bowl of chili one lunch. Every other breakfast, lunch, and dinner were combinations of red grapefruits, boiled eggs, raw spinach, boiled split peas, or grilled onions. And water of course. My food costs averaged just $4.75 daily.

Exercise facts

Total miles/kilometers walked or ellipsed: 191.25/307.79, daily average = 3.83/6.16

The number of weight training sessions: 20

Various core, leg, and arm exercises with free weights or nautilus machines, or simply pushups or sit ups on the floor.

Now it's one thing to lose weight quickly, as Method Three shows. It's quite another thing to do that *and* achieve *physical fitness personal bests (PB's)* at the same time. If both can be achieved at the same time, Method Three appears to a layman to be solid evidence that dietary choices are not only important but essential to a thriving, healthy body. Let's look at the PB's carved out in the *rope pull,* demonstrating incremental improvements from workout to workout, from Feb. 1, 2012 to Mar. 21, 2012.

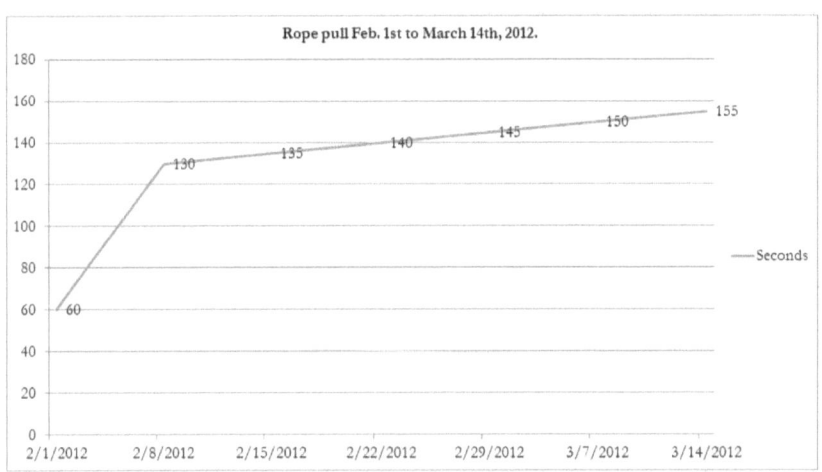

OK, 60 seconds, where I started, was actually too low in the body "taxing" department. So we see a steep jump to 130 seconds on Feb. 8. The gains from there to March 14, 2012 were incremental.

(And they felt inexorable too. Fast forward to March 4, 2013: my PB rope pull equals six minutes, 5 seconds or 365 seconds!)

Now let's take the bench press. With Method One, I had no spotter to ensure that I was not risking injury, so I did not do any bench presses. But from Methods Two through Four I did have a spotter. My progress in strength, while nothing to write home about, is something to write about here, to bear witness that your body will let you know if your diet and lifestyle changes are not only becoming a habit but slimming you down .

As you can see, there's been a dramatic improvement in the amount lifted—and all this while I was getting older, obviously. True, I can only do one repetition at 185 pounds (83.91 kg), but I see no reason why I should not be able to push 200 up there by, say, next year. As it turns out, on March 17th, 2013 I was able to bench 200 pounds (90.7 kg) for the first time. Enough about me. I'm just like you. You could achieve a similar gain in performance in an appropriate exercise, boosted by diet, given time, patience, and a stick-to-it attitude—and a spotter!

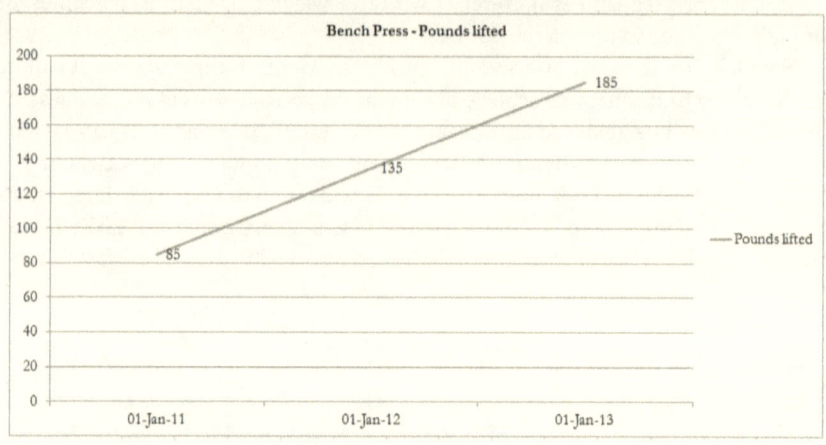

188.8 lbs 3 Feb 2012 / 185.6 lbs 6 Feb 2012 / 182.2 lbs 9 Feb 2012

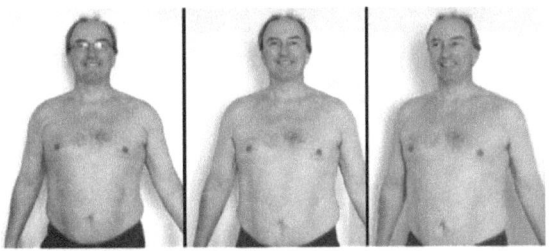

180.8 lbs 12 Feb 2012 / 178 lbs 15 Feb 2012 / 175.6 lbs 22 Feb 2012

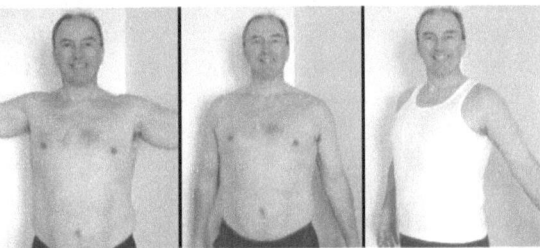

170.8 lbs 29 Feb 2012 / 166.8 lbs 9 March 2012 / 160.6 lbs 21 March 2012

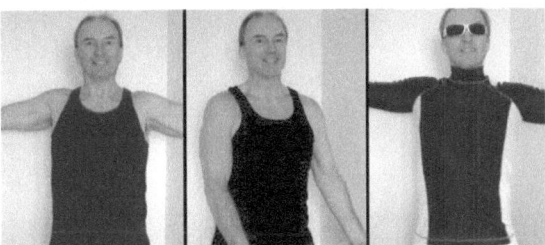

Method Three demonstrates the power of dietary choices as crucial to big time, quick time, weight loss. Consider that with Method Two I averaged 10+ miles (16.09+ kilometers) daily, whether on the elliptical or walking. Yet I lost much more weight daily with Method Three, and walked, or used the elliptical less than 4 miles (6.44 kilometers) per day. And the weight training exertions for Methods Two and Three were roughly equal. It was the *Fantastic Five foods factor*! You can see the difference in calories burned here:

Daily					
Method 2		Method 3		Method 3 – Method 2	
Pounds	Calories	Pounds	Calories	Caloric difference	
0.353	1,236	0.72	2,520	1,285	

Basically, because of the fantastic five foods, I dropped an extra 1,285 calories daily with method 3.

With five foods either boiled or eaten raw, simplicity and felicity were never very far away. My energy level was up and my workouts were never better.

Because Method Three has such a strong dietary change component, let's pick our forks at a couple of popular diet plans and a potentially amazing supplement. But first, a little jab back, via the strawberry, at all the pressure we feel to "go green and eat green." This pressure can become a distraction from our main goals.

Chapter 20
Food choices and your environment

A while back, I saw plastic packages of strawberries, of identical size, for sale at the supermarket. The ones grown locally in Ontario, a few blocks from where I lived at the time, cost $3.99 per pack. The ones from California, also grown locally a few thousand miles away, cost $1.99. Given that California grows the vast majority of strawberries in the USA, you gotta figure some are grown in Ontario, California.

Anyhow, I bought the latter pack. I love the earth and would love my local farmer if I ever met one. But I love my wallet, and I love my wallet fat with bills saved by buying food from growers in far-away lands. I gather I am supposed to loathe them for their effrontery and gall to allow their foods to get caught up in the military-industrial-complex-multinational-corporation-food-chain-distribution and retribution cycle.

A friendly piece of advice: If the goal is to lose weight through diet change, avoid getting caught up in a variety of unrelated food causes. You could end up doing everything except losing weight and helping everyone but yourself. So I don't feel too guilty about my food choice. In fact, I feel warm all over, knowing I might irk a tree hugger if I told one of my reprehensible buying habits.

But I'm gutless. If I am interrogated by some eco-nut, I'll adamantly aver that I only buy strawberries from Ontario.

Chapter 21
Dr. Moreno 17 day diet

It's hard to keep quiet about the Dr. Moreno 17 Day Diet. The diet industry is panting, his admirers are praising, while experts are wondering if his diet program—four cycles of 17 days each—lives up to the hype.

So what's the roar about? Try this on for size: Drop a dress size during the first 17 days, or the equivalent of 10–12 pounds lost, your choice.

It all comes down to choice of foods. And no, as Dr. Mike Moreno says, this isn't a feel good, happy-go-lucky diet; it takes discipline. It doesn't, fortunately or unfortunately, dig into deep-rooted emotional factors behind binge eating but deals with facts—cold hard facts, and lots of them.

Where does exercise kick in? Daily. For 17 minutes. Walking will do just fine, Dr. Moreno says, striking a "careful balance" between food and exercise. Push-ups aren't necessary. The 17 minutes per day of "easy" exercise is an easy number to remember, and easy enough on your body that it won't get trashed like it did back in the '70's under the high impact maxim and mantra of "No pain, no gain."

When can you "pig out" again? Unlike "The 4-Hour Body," the best seller written by Tim Ferriss which offers a cheat day, Dr. Moreno doesn't counsel picking a day to hang around your favorite buffet morning, noon, and night. Within the 4th cycle some naughty foods are allowed, on weekends.

Can one partake of spirits? The 17 Day Diet advises dieters to avoid alcohol during the initial stages.

Isn't this just a rehash of diet books of yore? Some feel it is the Atkins diet revisited. But most of the feedback from lay reviewers leans to laudatory spins, advertising their personal "get small" triumphs throughout Twitter, YouTube, and the blogosphere at large.

Chinese philosopher Confucius proverbed: A journey of a thousand miles begins with a single step. The first step in the opening 17-day cycle is the biggest step, with the most restrictive daily intake of 1,200 calories kicking in.

Hands up—who is Dr. Mike Moreno? First and foremost, he is a family doctor. He says 80% of his new patients are overweight.

How, in a nutshell, does the 17 Day Diet get you small? The 17-day cycles are a process but all stages have one overarching principle: to purge the system of processed foods in favor of natural foods. We know that makes eminent sense; we've heard time and time again—shop in the supermarket's outside aisles where the fresh fruit, vegetables, meats, and fish are offered; we know that junk food has such colorful packaging, with prizes offered to the tots, mainly because the contents are, well, junk; we know, or surmise, that what Dr. Moreno is telling us really isn't new. But the pitch, that is, the results of his program in dropping 10–12 pounds in just 17 days, is new. Any way you slice it.

He does give the crossed-fingers-behind-the-back disclaimer, in reference to his own patients' experience with the diet (i.e., results can vary). But everyone disclaims the heck out of everything they write and do these days, so that's par for the course.

He does, however, hack and slice away at the opinions of those who scoff that much of the initial weight loss is water. So what, he answers: weight is weight, water or otherwise. As a side benefit, much of the water excreted will be old water, which has been stored and sloshing around the hips and thighs.

Dr. Moreno was interviewed by Dr. Phil, and many others besides, and he stresses that the 17 Day Diet is not gimmicky or faddish. Rather, he believes, it's a life changer, a guide to how one can, if the diet is adopted, live in a healthy way forever. As for the 17 days? He says: "Anybody can do everything for 17 days, it's a soft number."

But, forever is a hard number, and a long time. Will this diet drop that waistline and raise that self-esteem, like now? Possibly, if you follow the instructions to a "T." But know that, for the USA alone, all the T's are crossed and the I's are dotted. According to a Marketdata Enterprises market report for 2010, those who produce books and tapes for the self-help weight-loss industry are endorsing checks expected to bring in *13.9 billion.* So Dr. Moreno has lots of competition from weight loss theorists offering a variety of programs, many promising weight loss on easier terms.

Yet Dr. Moreno's 17 Day Diet has been first in line at the cashiers.

Chapter 22
The Dukan diet

The Dukan Diet is worth reading up on. The creator, Dr. Pierre Dukan, dares us: will that be vegetables or the gastric band? First, let's get to the meat of the matter, besides the protein: The Dukan diet has wowed France for 10 years and now happily threatens to parlay America's waistlines to, well, less wide than they are now.

Are any Americans listening? Kate Middleton, rumor has it, used this diet before her wedding. Jennifer Lopez, rumors report, also uses it.

Unlike the Dr. Moreno 17 Day Diet, which is organized into cycles, Dr. Dukan's diet has phases, four of them. There are some similarities however: Both diets eschew junk food, and both tout walking as the key exercise component. But the protein mix is quite different. In phase one—the Attack phase— Dr. Dukan's diet features only low fat proteins, oat bran, and water. And whereas in Dr. Moreno's diet, the first three cycles of four last 17 days each, Dr. Dukan's second phase— the Cruise phase—can last months. Phase three is Consolidation. Phase four, Stabilization, lasts a lifetime if all goes well.

Both diets offer big weight loss benefits in their first stages. Possibly pare 7–10 pounds in five days with the Dukan diet; move 10–12 pounds off that frame in just 17 days with the Moreno.

If you are using the Dukan diet, stick with the color green, as vegetables go. Forego the orange of carrots and the yellow of corn. Water is de rigueur and even coffee is passable, so long as it is mixed with water, and not milk, cream, or sugar.

Five million French can't be wrong. At least, that's what the book blazons on its cover. And whether this claim represents the success of five million French at shedding the avoirdupois or is just a puff number plucked out of who knows where, Dr. Dukan's own theories didn't come from the dark side of the moon. He says he studied 210 diets and interviewed countless people of all walks (and shapes) of life. He sounds pretty well grounded when he claims that humans use food for a crutch, for comfort, for credibility—for a cornucopia of circumstances. Even titans, people who have reached the pinnacle of success, crumble and quake, surrendering all discipline—slavering when they view a favorite food or a potential feast.

As a nutritionist for over 30 years, Dr. Dukan has been writing and spreading the good word, and he has made his mark. Now his followers, in more than 100 online forums ("dukanons"), pick up any slack. "Dukanettes" often blog their experiences with weight loss. No doubt the fact that he is a nutritionist serves Dr. Dukan well. A nutritionist's sole focus is teaching and promoting healthy eating habits. Think of a cheerleader with a spoon and spatula, instead of pom-poms.

Dr. Dukan, despite his credentials, is above all, deep down, a realist; he says only you can do it. Only you can ultimately lose whatever weight you want to. No one else. Despite his best efforts and his team of specialists, he admits that the subject must play the leading role in losing the largeness.

But he *can* help customize and tailor your progress specifically to your personality. This he does via *The Book of My Weight,* which is not so much a book as a program and an analysis fitted for each and every one who undertakes the regimen, to make sure that lost weight stays lost.

How? 154 ways, that's how. Each person, he maintains, is unique. No argument there. As such, we each have our own individual gourmet-grazing-gormandizing patterns, and our own "weight personality." To bolster his point (and our uniqueness) he has 154 questions about food for the reader to answer.

The gazillions of possible answers to the 154 queries assign every reader a specific genetic eating code—which results in a not-off-the-rack, not-another-cookie-cutter weight loss book unique to the reader. It can be used to successfully lose and keep that weight off, through lifestyle changes.

Lifestyle changes? Pick a diet, any diet. Dr. Dukan asserts that *any* diet can make you lose weight—in the short term. But in the long term? Nope. Not unless your root causes for rushing, raiding, and rifling the refrigerator are probingly, painstakingly, and particularly assessed and assayed.

Clearly, not a canned conclusion.

And don't look for canned foods in his diet either. Look for proteins, 72 of them, plus 28 types of vegetables. These form the bulwark and backbone of allowable foods in the Dukan diet.

Contrary to most diet counselors, Dr. Dukan *does* allow this, the "six magic words": 'EAT AS MUCH AS YOU WANT!'

Which would seem to run counter to his argument that an overabundance of food in our developed nations leads to obesity. Indeed, obesity is no "fat" joke. The World Health Organization (WHO) calls obesity in the Western world the "first non-infectious epidemic." Clearly, the epidemic must be treated. Is the Dukan diet a wise prescription?

Remember, we were told that five million French can't be wrong. Can't they? Could those 100-plus online fan forums following Dr. Dukan's diet and dissertations be deceiving themselves but no one else? Can one really eat as much as one wants? If only to check out that last point, for that reason alone, it might be worth the money to spring for the book and give it a good, long, serious look.

Chapter 23

Moringa oleifera—Nature's perfect supplement?

Supplement this! You could do tons worse than adding Moringa oleifera to your recipe, regimen, and repertoire. Any way you slice it, cut it, chop it, or analyze it, Moringa—a vegetable tree—packs a punch way above its planetary weight.

Consider, comparing apples to apples, in this case gram for gram or ounce for ounce, the extremely nutritious leaves. These powerhouses have been shown by research to pack more Vitamin C than oranges, more potassium than bananas, three times the iron of spinach, four times the calcium in milk, and more Vitamin A than carrots.

These are not made-up, hocus pocus, feel-good flimflammery findings about the vegetable-of-the-month either. Nutritional science is taking notice. The National Institutes for Health has taken a shine to Moringa, naming it the Plant of the Year in 2008. And the tree attached to those leaves is a very hardy beast, tolerating lousy soil and paltry amounts of rain. Even the roots rock: they are full of water to help the plant through long dry periods.

Hardy and healthy. And handy. The leaves, in a pinch, can be ground up and used to clean knives and forks—and walls. Or you can sprinkle ground-leaf powder as a spice on a meal, your call.

Heck, even the creamy, yellow-white flowers are edible. And good for you too.

But the Moringa won't clean the fridge. Which is somehow fitting, given that the leaves can be left outside to the elements in powder form—for months—without losing any of their nutritional value. Given that the developing world, or Third World, is developing a first class case of soaring obesity rates, the Moringa sounds like the perfect "fit" antidote to the fat spread.

But today, it's all about you, and you ail putridly; your doctor, specialist, and quack cousin have diagnosed you with diabetes, HIV, an ulcer, lotsa tumors, a wonky prostate, menstrual problems (if relevant) arthritis, and acne. And the quack cousin discerned all this from reading your palm.

No sweat. No sweaty palms either. Know why? Because the Moringa oleifera is reputed to prevent and treat these eight calamity diseases, and another 292 besides. An even 300. Wow.

Not surprisingly, eastern medicine specialists from India, where this tree originally made itself at home in the foothills of the Himalayas, have had the time and patience, through Ayurvedic medicine, to learn of its dietary and health benefits.

Say you don't live in India, but you really want to go au naturel, back to the earth, and live like your great-grandparents did, assuming they could have had lighting and heating. You could buy Moringa seeds (don't cheat and eat 'em fresh or roast 'em up when they age) and plant them indoors. They'll germinate at around 70 degrees Fahrenheit. You can also propagate from limb cuttings.

In your backyard "back forty," if you prune the branches from this fast-growing tree judiciously, throughout the year, you can get about *nine harvests*. How's about them apples?

There's more good growing news. For farmers in the southern Philippines or the Visayas region, where farming is perennially tough (like everywhere else) and cash crop prices are an annual guessing ordeal, some are considering Moringa as a revenue producer, because the plant can also be used as a biofuel.

Cool.

Let's say you hate gardening, and your green thumbs are actually green painted concrete—concrete you wish to pave your-soon-to-be ex-spouse's vegetable-patch over with. Here too, the Moringa seeds can help. While pouring all the concrete, and sweating up a storm, simply grind up those seeds and use them to purify the water you'll be gulping down.

And unlike the marijuana leaf or bud, which is of medical use in reducing nausea and glaucoma (but can induce paranoia), the Moringa leaf, when not feeding the family, can also embellish your soul and system by beautifying the skin, nourishing the brain, and yes, promoting energy. All the while it helps digestion and aids the circulatory system also. Oh yeah, in its spare time, it puts on its Superman cape and helps care for the immune system and - irons out those wrinkles.

Not only is it versatile in benefits, it's got a whole bunch of names to boot. How about the Clarifier tree, the Horseradish tree, or the Drumstick tree?

OK, there has to be an "on the other hand," a downside, a negative right? What are its drawbacks? Hmmm. It won't send you screaming into the night scouring the landscape for a substance abuse retreat. It won't rot your liver like booze. It won't coagulate your lungs like hydroponic killer reefer.

According to a Discovery Channel documentary, Moringa is also known as a "miracle tree." In Africa it could be the bulwark against malnutrition. In Senegal, they swear by it. Or at least bless it.

Everybody under the sun with propeller heads and thinking caps is researching the merits of Moringa, including the National Geographic Society, and the Andrew Mellon foundation, to name but two high-forehead institutions. In India, for example, there are a lot of blind people. Researchers are looking at the Moringa, with its loads of Vitamin A, as a possible weapon in the fight against lost sight.

And that is the long and short of it. Powerful in nutrition and near magical in medicine, simple to prepare and easy to use, the Moringa tree seems absolutely perfect as a remedy or a building block, for you or for me, to rebuild or create from new—a strong, sustainable, healthy society. We need more of these kinds of solutions.

Now on to Method Four: I stopped weighing myself. But there's way more. Read on.

Chapter 24
Why method four? For a healthy you with a no pressure exercise and eating program

Method Four: Weights and Walking but no Weigh-ins

Of course, "no pressure" doesn't mean "anything goes." A healthy you still means no junk food, alcohol, or cigarettes. But stay tuned.

Method Four, which officially started on the July 1st 2012, has no starting picture. Why? Simply because we've seen that scene before with Methods One through Three. And also because the first picture I remembered to take was at the Calgary Stampede on July 7th. The coat I was wearing concealed the rounded contours and soft shoulders underneath. Yes, I thought a bulky coat would hide the bulky body. I had gained back all the weight that I had lost with Method Three to the tune of about 190 pounds. I looked sloppy, slouchy, slovenly.

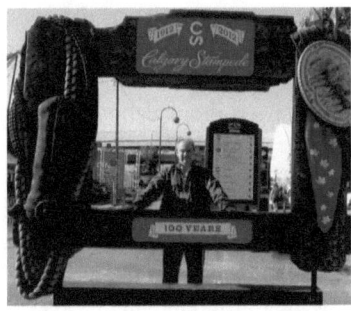

And grouchy. Unless you want to write a book extolling the merits(?) of losing and gaining weight more often than Madonna changes sartorial styles, don't do what I did. It can't be stressed enough just how awful it is to go from fat to fit, to fat to fit, to fat to fit, to fat to fit. So this was it. I made a conscious decision to never gain back that weight. I expect my weight to vary from day to day, what with water retention, the occasional buffet binge-out, holiday-vacation meals, and so on. The reason I feel confident that I can keep my weight down anyway is primarily due to one factor.

Honesty.

I have been brutally honest with myself. Every time I purposely gained the weight back, I did so by eating healthy meals topped off with loads of junk food. And I knew I'd be kidding myself if I thought I could reintroduce junk food into my menu because I don't do "casual" junk food well. I love the stuff even more than I hate the inevitable crash and burn, with sugar levels rising and dropping faster than a kid on a pogo stick. So I have stricken it from my life. I had proven, time and time again, that I do not have enough discipline or self-control to avoid gobbling up goodies while watching the boob tube at night.

So how's that junk food ban working out, you may ask, and how, specifically, did I do it? Well so far it's working out just fine. Since July 1st of 2012, I have had but one dessert, and that was on Christmas Day of that year. I have not had a craving for the sweet or salty stuff before or after, save for one instance I'll explain later. Now, to stay on the wagon, I had to take some proactive measures. I keep my head down when whooshing through junk-food aisles in supermarkets. When I watch TV at night, I must contend with all those execrable food ads. But, by and large, my success in shunning such foods comes down to motivation and proof. I've proven I can gain lots of weight with junk food, whether intentionally or not. If I wanted to keep the weight off, and write a book showing that weight could be kept off, then I had better walk the walk and prove that a life without sweets, excess salt, high fats, and lots of additives is both possible and pleasant.

Specifically, I have replaced junk foods with good foods that I love, and I don't stint on the number of meals daily, or the portions. On the weekend I might have five to six meals Saturday and Sunday, as opposed to the three meals I have Monday to Friday. I have found eating a big breakfast is a huge boon to avoiding the need to snack at night. To reinforce that habit, I now usually wake up an hour earlier and go to bed an hour earlier that I have ever done before. And I must add that I purged all liquids from my diet except for water. Water is the only liquid one needs to maintain health, and assist weight loss. That, plus saying no to junk food, has given me more energy.

Much more energy. I now need about an hour to an hour and a half less sleep per night. Basically, my meals are about 70% protein. Protein "fills one up." That percentage may not work for you because of preference or health issues. But whatever you eat must help you curb the hanky panky, that is, wanting to wantonly raid the fridge or pantry for any bad foods that may be lurking there.

You must eat enough of whatever's right for you, so you don't feel you are missing out or sacrificing life's little enjoyments that come with dining. I would venture to say that as you lose weight and still satisfy your dietary needs and lusts, you'll feel that you've gained—gained power to control what you eat, the power of self-confidence and the power of a healthier body. Subtracting junk food from your life can be a huge plus.

So honesty, in unabashedly reviewing my relationship with junk food was, and is, critical.

Adaptability will come in very handy too because if you want to curb junk foods, or pub food, or that donut with the morning coffee, you might have to watch from the sidelines while your friends partake. You can joke with them, saying that you are their escort, ensuring nothing gets out of hand. That gives you the perfect excuse to remain vigilant, unencumbered by snacking and sipping—and if they are good colleagues or buddies, they should not mind your changed behavior. If, after some initial razzing, they persist in pestering you about your stoicism in the face of coffee shop treats, you might want to shop for some new friends, or at least go out with the current ones less often. Or, give them this line: "I seem to be losing my taste for sweets." (Many of us will more readily accept the excuse of mere preference than a conscious vote for better health, because it does not induce a guilt trip!)

Similarly, eating meals with family might mean arranging for your meals to be prepared separately, befitting your new choices. This will go down a lot easier with others if you prepare your eats yourself, and clean up afterwards.

Here's what I did, and did not do, in Method Four.

Method	4
Smoking	N
Alcohol	N**
Junk food	N
Walking	Y
Elliptical	Y
Weight training	Y
Tracking process	Y
Weigh ins – scale	N
Fitness trainer	N
Pounds lost	35* (kg = 15.87)
Time taken	215 days
Average pounds lost per day	0.163
Average grams lost per day	73.94

For method 4 the 35 pounds dropped happened between July 1, 2012 and January 31, 2013. But method 4, with my final picture taken just before this book went to print, officially ended June 30, 2013. ** Unofficially I will be thriving by method 4 for the rest of my life, save for imbibing with friends once in a while. It is, by far, the easiest to maintain for diet, yet improve for fitness levels, of all the four methods.

And a new chrome dome.

I have to admit I did bend to peer pressure and had a sip of moonshine and about a half a beer with co-workers at a dinner party, Saturday Feb 23rd, 2013. Both the moonshine—made from grapes with a smell that would knock you over even before the alcohol swigged did—and the beer—tasted great. I wondered whether I could lean over the edge of the wagon, so to speak, and try to drink alcohol in moderation, while still holding off on the cigarettes?

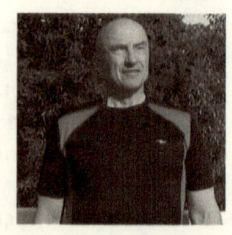

About two weeks later, on a Friday, I had two beers with co-workers, with no cigarettes, though later, on the train home, I felt a couple of pangs for a puff.

Honestly, I realized I would have to be *very careful* about putting myself in such a precariously tempting position—it would be too easy to want a cigarette after a few beers. But because I had had a tiny bit of booze in front of these friends from work, twice now, I hoped they would accept my attempt to meet them halfway. They won, I succumbed—but in the long run I've won, if they, and I, can now turn our attention to other matters.

Method Four featured a key qualitative difference from the others methods. I never weighed myself, or thought of doing so, save for Jan. 31st 2013 when I stepped on the scales, noting my 35 pound drop. How I kept track of the weight loss was by sight and feel. For sight, I'd look at myself in the mirror and grunt or grin, depending on what I saw. For feel, I felt how tight my pants were around the waist. If I took 20 minutes of tugging and rolling around the floor to hike the blue jeans up, I knew I was not ready for that waist size. Gradually I got down to a 30-inch (76 centimeter) waist for pants. Now, having been down there a few months, I know that if the pants are starting to feel a little snug (that is, if I start swooning and fainting from the shortage of oxygen to my brain), I have undoubtedly added a few pounds to my frame. So I cut back meal portion sizes, especially chicken wings—a top food favorite of mine—and mushroom soup, and eat more of the five foods I used exclusively in Method Three (red grapefruit, onions, spinach, split pea legumes, and eggs).

Generally, however, I tinker with portions. I haven't had to excise any healthy edibles. In fact, since I don't eat lousy foods I have often added new foods to my menu. I'm sure you've read elsewhere that adding new foods to your diet causes your body to react favorably because it's getting variety, not getting too comfortable with the same old, same old. So when my pants wear tight, I have added pork and steak as alternatives to my main dinner protein of chicken.

Not weighing myself certainly lowered the stress level. No longer a prisoner to the daily or weekly emotional highs or bluesy lows that inevitably come from reading the scale, I could go about my business on an even keel. I did not feel under pressure to lose that extra pound pronto, nor was I beset by undue depression if my weight had increased two days in a row. How many of us, having had an unfavorable or unexpected weigh-in result, have then gone off the deep end and pigged out on bad foods, or gone on a booze blast to compensate? Most of us, right?

Speaking of deep ends, how do you feel about birthdays and getting older? I just had one… If you can't take stock of your situation on a birthday, when can you?

Chapter 25
56th Birthday

You only get one totally personal and poignant kick at the can each year to reflect on what's gone on and what's gone wrong, and how you plan to fix the latter. This is what birthdays are for. If you are young and lucky, it's cake and ice cream. If you are like most of us older folk, it feels like just deserts, no matter if you've been bad or good. I am firmly in middle age now, for better or for worse, and that's the perfect time to examine one's achievements and failures with an unbiased, even a jaundiced, eye.

Why?

Well because only the jerks in your life will tell you you're a flop on your big day. People might even try to be nice and compliment you when no such accolades are deserved. So it's up to you to determine if your goals have been realistic, if you've gone a long way toward meeting them, or have fallen far short. And whether your plan to fix your failings is at all realistic.

So you contemplate and consider…

56 years old today. And no junk food for the past seven months. Don't miss that stuff, but I'd sure like a spin at being 20 something again!

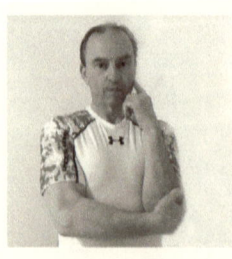 I contemplated becoming melancholy, wistfully ruing the years gone by, and the times wasted doing boom all. But I flung the angst out the window in favor of a jolt, a pick-me-up, a gentlemen start-your-engines boost, courtesy of my first cup of coffee *ever*. I had sat on the sidelines for 55 years and 364 days, and now was the time to check out this coffee thing. Was it just today's fad that might last as long as tomorrow, if the masses took to it?

Let me tell you, I began to think coffee may be here to stay. And it was hard for me to explain at the time because I was stuck to the ceiling, higher than a kite, and more jittery than a waterbug.

Yes, that was after three lattes with a shot of espresso in each, at no charge thanks to my friends at work who wanted to watch my ensuing antics. Rather than muse over a life somewhat well lived, I just wanted to see the next daybreak, free from the shakes and quakes. Land sakes, that birthday coffee spree set me in a hornet's nest brew stew, light years from a calm, cool, and collected composure.

Good to know. But I'm a slow learner. The next time I whirl into the coffee maelstrom full bore will be when I turn 112, with six cups. As any addict will tell you: Anything worth doing is worth overdoing... six cups should be enough.

In the meantime I realized I had better get back on the beam and finish off Method Four. I had planned to peak around June 2013 and caffeine wasn't part of the program. Now that I recall the episode, that was the first time anything liquid but water had passed my lips since July 1, 2012.

The next day, I returned to my normal (crazy) self. Life has gotten in the way of the best laid plans of mice and men again...

Chapter 26
Falling off the wagon, hard. (Actually, it was easy)

Oh god, my life was over. I had received bad news from work. I won't go into details about the news. But I can tell you how I reacted. So what did I do? I decided I'd show 'em, show 'em what I'm made of. I left work early, came home, and started my sorry sob story by cracking open three tins of iced tea and one V-8. And don't I feel great?

I feel like shit. And it's not so much because I've betrayed the water diet I've been on since July 1st, 2012, but because of how the sugar in the drinks has made my throat dry and my forehead sweaty. My stomach was a-rumble, and my life a-tumble. Downwards.

Except I've learned one thing. Two things actually. First of all, I learned, for the mequillionth time, that when I face an obstacle, I'm not above putting myself behind the eight-ball in screwing myself over, for reasons only god knows why. I am often my own worst enemy. Secondly, and this is kind of a new revelation (or at least one I had forgotten), the sugar high and taste, while sweet, is fleeting. I looked forward to the next day when I could get back to water only. *Every time* I drink water, I sigh with contentment. My swigs of these liquids left me groaning with resentment. Big difference.

I would like to have said, "We now bring you back to our regularly scheduled program. Just had to get this off my chest." But I had to go because there was still a half-can of ice tea to knock back. I sensed that my self-destruction mode would not be over until I could feel the liquids swooshing sickly in my stomach. You have to hit rock bottom before you can come back, right?

Two days later I bought two bags of Jalapeño chips, a jug of 3.25% homogenized milk, and a bottled milk shake—370 calories worth of thick goo that would hardly go down the gullet. Polished off the milkshake and about 2 glasses of milk, and about half a bag of chips. I was hoping I would throw out the other bag of chips and pour out the rest of the milk.

A couple of days later, I finished off the milk, but still had not opened the other bag of chips. One out of two isn't bad. And I didn't feel overly guilty. I wasn't going to jump off a bridge or anything. Because Method Four is an exercise and diet program that is eminently livable, it can withstand some side journeys into dumb dietary choices. And where was I on June 30, 2013, the official end of Method 4? I had not had junk food for weeks. As for liquids, for the past few weeks prior to June 30th it had been water only, except for drinks with friends in two instances, one jug of milk, and one jug of juice.

But now, how about we put me aside for a moment and look at what's happening today in the world of fat vs. fit, a world in which you must make your way toward the healthiest possible you.

First, we'll look at sports that amateurs can easily learn and practice at a variety of fitness levels ("Fitness for health well into old age"). Not everyone can lift weights, but the good news is, you don't have to. You just have to keep up the sports that you enjoy, that are right for you. Along the way, we will look at some surprising fat-to-fit struggles of pro athletes. Yes, *pro athletes*. Forget the hype; they have the same struggles as you and me. After that, we will look at some sports choices and stories that are a bit off the beaten track, but worth knowing about. They may spark some new ideas. We should all exercise our imaginations more.

Many people think that smoking or other substance use, or radical methods such as surgery, help weight control, so we had better have a look at those topics. ("Does smoking or other substance use help or hurt weight control?" and "Giving nature a nudge—is it worth the risks?")

Okay, so there is the challenge of getting the weight off, and then there is the challenge of *keeping* it off. In "Work and school fitness," we'll have a look at how to stay fit despite the fact that both work and school these days tend to mean a lot of sitting down.

And if we choose to just abandon our own health, wouldn't you know, in the age of free public health care, it turns out that the government is happy to try slimming us down via new rules and regulations ("Governments declare war on obesity"). It probably works about as well as most government crusades. That said, obesity *is* a genuine problem, and one that is beginning to affect children ("Fat jokes shouldn't be for kids").

After we take a look, just for fun, at some really extreme sports, we will close with a look at some obesity myths that are dead and, we hope, buried. And here's to your best health!

But before we plunge in, let's take a moment to savor Toronto's Mayor Ford's war on fat. Say what you want about the guy, unlike some other politicians these days, he is not trying to forcibly slim *you* down, he took on the challenge for himself. How did he do?

Part Two

Chapter 27
Toronto Mayor Rob Ford—Cut the waist challenge

Toronto mayor Rob Ford is a menace to himself and a total anchor on his wife and kids. For other children and casual observers he's a head scratcher, for fans in Ford Nation he's a delight, and for the media he's a dream. It isn't often that a completely calamitous typhoon like typhoon Haiyan, that smashed the Philippines, has to share the world spotlight and be nearly crowded out by the larger-than-life blowhard hiz-zoner, but it happened. Now that we adults have all had a refresher in the devilish doings of Rob Ford with (or without) escorts, crack, P---y, and a defamation lawsuit almost filed by Star reporter Daniel Dale, and this was written December 20, 2013, God knows what he's been up to, or down to since then – here's the piece below when all Rob Ford was concerned about - was losing weight. (Oh, by the way, Ford may be a boob and a bumpkin to some, but his bobblehead dolls are selling quicker than a horse tail flicks flies.)

Is your mayor a fathead? Is he or she also a fatty generally? Toronto mayor Rob Ford admits he's the latter, and detractors swear he's the former too.

What to do?

Smarten up? No can do, his opponents fret and fume. They bellow that Ford is a fellow incapable of the intellectual heavy lifting needed to look at issues free from ingrained bias—in other words, to see the issues as they do. And so, they charge, he's diverting attention from his "disastrous" first term as mayor by carping that he and everyone within earshot should lose weight.

Full disclosure: Ford's gigantic. But perhaps this suits him, given that Toronto is the hugest city in Canada. He has admitted to being disgusted with himself. Whether he's dramatizing his own problems in order to turn voters' attentions away from the monstrous problems that beset Toronto or sincere in spreading a good health message by spreading himself thin, one thing's for sure: Toronto and its mayor have lotsa waste and lotsa waist.

Rob Ford looks like the driver of the getaway car with a mug only a pug could love and an attitude akin to a rat's ass, only more voluble. Many folks love him. Just as many loathe him. There is no middle ground with this guy, save for that vast middle ground around his middle.

Before Ford became obsessed with physical fat, he ranted on about political fat. During the 2010 mayoral campaign, he promised to cut the fat at City Hall and slice and dice the fat-cat union "jobs for life" mentality that has pervaded the "Big Smoke" since who knows when. But now...

Rob Ford, as of 16 January 2012, waddled onto the scales at 330 pounds. The public name of the brothers' Ford official weight loss gauntlet was: Cut the Waist Challenge! Every Monday morning there was an official weigh-in to determine whether Ford was putting his money, and no junk food, where his mouth was. His Web site, cutthewaist.ca (no longer on line as of March 2013) said that he and his councilor brother Doug, who's also a political porker, each lost 16 pounds. Doug initially tipped the scales at 275 pounds.

Down 16 flabby pounds in just over two weeks? Not too shabby for the self-described "300 pounds of fun." Mayor Rob Ford attributes his about-face to find the thin within to an epiphany. He woke up one morning and realized that he had young kids. Kids like to play. Especially with a dad who's alive.

One of Ford's faux pas has been binging on ice cream late at night. Admittedly, it's not as bad as alcohol, but February 2nd, 2012, the Internet and newspapers screamed headlines about sugar as a toxic substance that should be kept from, or rationed to, the little ones.

I hope Rob Ford will eventually lose serious weight and gain the energy he will need to hector recalcitrant council members. He'll be able to fight the good fight harder and longer against his inveterate media enemy, the *Toronto Star*. He might attend parades; the *Star* gave a "gotcha" to Ford for not bowing down to the gay community when he didn't watch their more edgy parade partakers prance in their gotchies. (In 2013, he partially fixed this shortcoming, attending the raising of the rainbow flag, setting off Pride Week events.)

Left-wingers won't be happy if Ford sticks with the diet and sticks with living for a while. They'd like him gone, like yesterday. Maybe not deader than a doornail, but at least buried six feet under politically.

Rob Ford is an impolitic politician. He has been about as politically correct as the Hunchback of Notre Dame has been erect, which is to say, not at all. He extols trucks—and excoriates cyclists—and has too much chutzpah to boot. In daring North American mayors to shape up or ship out, he caught New York City mayor Bloomberg in his net. Bloomberg, however, is one svelte puppy, even if he whines a lot.

Other mayors, like Calgary's Naheed Nenshi for example, are taking a hands-off approach to Ford's overture.

Rob's a pro-car guy all the way, so he won't go completely off the deep end and start advocating for the survival of the earth, but he will fight for his own survival.

It's the least he could do, and darn it, he's going to do it. Besides, it's a lot more fun than trying to right, and run, a city as dysfunctional as Toronto. As a councilor, Ford dipped into his own pockets to pay his office expenses instead of milking the taxpayer as is legally mandated in "Hogtown," and was investigated by the city's integrity commissioner for his trouble.

Not surprisingly, a guy as big as Ford is a man of many talents. Besides being a right-wing bloviator, he blows the whistle, coaching the Don Bosco Catholic

Secondary School football team. But, as of May 2013, Toronto's Catholic school board has axed Ford as that team's coach.

Losing weight—especially fat—is not easy, as about 112% of the world's population knows. But here's one thing we all know: By making your get-fit goals public, and measureable, your chances of success are immensely increased.

So Ford's not all talk. He's walking the walk. And if he can lose the weight as rapidly as he seems to have lost his mind, what with his one-track approach to all things subway, as opposed to Light Rapid Transit, Ford will be fit, right quick.

Rob Ford is not only trimming fat by cutting back sugar, he's paring his entitlements fat, cutting back lucre. He intends to forego the 2012 cost-of-living increase allocated to Toronto councilors. He's hoping other politicians will follow his financial weight loss example.

He had also hoped to be down 50 pounds by June 18th, 2012. He didn't make it, not by a country mile, losing a relatively paltry 17 pounds, finishing up at 313 pounds. To add insult to injury, he twisted his ankle as he stepped off the scale. You can't make this stuff up. As to how Rob Ford, who wanted to shed 50 pounds, will make up the 33 pound difference, is anybody's guess. Don't hold your breath.

But don't count him out either. This guy's always up to something.

Chapter 28
Pilates: What's it all about?

Fitness for the Healthiest Possible You—Now and Onward

On Valentine's Day I hoped to find true love in the afternoon with Pilates. I had a 30 minute complimentary session, a taste test so to speak, and a one-on-one with Kathy (not her real name) in the studio. She was to teach me a little about this workout I know so little about. Here's what happened:

I was 40 minutes early. I had a steam and headed to the gym where I loosened up further with the few Yoga moves that I remembered and could still do. Then I headed to the health club computers where I read up on the net about Joseph Pilates and how he developed his exercise program. Disciplined guy.

"Studio," as in Pilates Studio, seems a tad presumptuous as a name. It's nothing more than a square room with a floor and a door. But the door does have a little window. I, peeping Tom-style, peeked in. A sandy-haired wiry man, maybe fifty plus, was explaining something to a young woman. She was prone on what could be mistaken for an S&M contraption, except for the fact that it was lying on the floor and not chained to a wall.

Where was Kathy? I asked at the front desk. Generally fitness professionals are prompt. The guy manning the phones could not find her on the schedule so he left her a message to call me. I was bummed but took solace in the thought that at least I had tried. I did my part. It's not my fault. But I didn't take the extra step and mitigate my losses by asking the man teaching if he could take me through a few moves.

Case solved! The missing Pilates instructor wasn't missing at all. She offered up the feeble excuse that the Wednesday appointment—as etched in my brain—was actually set for Thursday at 3:00 PM. Her excuse was true. What's my excuse? Over-eager? Hyper-anxious? Inattentive to detail? Thick as a brick? Take your pick.

I got it right the next time and met Kathy, and she started by handing me a document. I looked at it and her, and she explained that it was a waiver, standard stuff, just saying I could not sue her brains out, should I hurt myself. That done, we began with some abdominal preparation work on a smooth orange surface mat. I learned orange is an "out there" mat color and mats, orange or not, are expensive. I also learned that six-pack muscles, the male, macho, masculine mountain of it all (something I, and most guys, hold dear even if we don't own a set) aren't the real deal. She agreed that they look great but added that they do diddly for core or stability.

There are, as it happens, four abdominal groups, the *transversus abdominus*, the *rectus abdominus*, the external oblique muscles, and the internal oblique muscles, none of which were firing on any cylinders for me. And I didn't know how to summon them to show up and do so. Apparently, the underlying layers of muscles make the difference in Pilates. And lying down and trying to activate muscles I didn't even know existed five minutes ago was frustrating. (I get the same frustrated feeling whenever I try to meditate. I just don't get it.)

Anyway, I wasn't getting these muscles to move. She exhorted me to inhale and exhale properly. I didn't realize there was a proper way. Shoulders off the floor, she continued, don't forget to relax the shoulders now, keep the palms of the hands parallel to the ceiling, don't forget to breathe, stand up, sit down, fight, fight, fight...

Not me. I was ready to throw in the towel. She said cranking up the layers of my abdominals would come. When? Not in this half hour, which was now down ten minutes, and I didn't know if I had accomplished anything—but my curiosity at my utter inability to probe the surface of Pilates was piqued.

Out of nowhere came a pink cue tip, as wide as a bucket and as tall as a barstool.

"Lie on this."

"Pardon?"

"Lie on this."

"On this?"

Yes, on that."

"What is—?"

"Sit on the end."

"Pardon?"

"Sit, put your bum on the end and shinny back."

"Right, then. I'll shinny back and do what?"

I had little composure and lousy posture—at least for Pilates. We were nearly out of time so we went back to talking about the four abdominal groups.

"What do you feel in your stomach?" she asked.

"I sense I'm feeling nearly something or other; when can I expect anything to happen? Actually I feel nothing."

I should have been grounded in the basics, having been schooled in assuming a neutral pelvic position. I could have grasped that the abdominals should be pulled down and into the mat. I could have weathered up to 100 arm pumps. Maybe I could have graduated to the roll up move, an all encompassing head-to-toe motion from a nearly outstretched body with the arms above the head at a 45 degree angle to a jackknife one. It looks smooth and soothing, but is probably harder to perform well than it appears...

I might have realized that the glowing testimonials Pilates' participants gave for its ability to reduce or eradicate prior back pains and poor posture were refreshingly heartfelt; they enthused over how it helped them with tough pregnancies and difficulties after childbirth. So many of them seemed to leave classes, at all levels of expertise, both free of tension and full of energy.

But I learned about the larger picture, if not the details. To get a feel of Pilates, one should probably start out with an introductory one-hour session, minimum. To get the hang of Pilates might take a long time, to master Pilates, a lifetime.

I didn't stick with it but I know I'll come back to it. I'm just not sure when. I think, however, that to have true core conditioning and control, I'll need all my abdominal "equipment" working for me. So I won't be face-to-face with a Pilates starter session again until after I watch a few videos of how it's actually done. That did not happen last Valentine's day (2013). I had a cold, the sniffles, a pressure-packed stuffed head and more aches and pains than a professional wrestler deprived of painkillers. But I was at least able to stretch that morning. Though it isn't Pilates, it did feel soothing, even for the scanty few minutes I lumbered around to limber up.

Chapter 29

Shakira takes up golf. Go fore it. We're for it.

Speaking of Limber...

Sexy, sultry, belly-dancing Shakira has a fire in her belly. For golf. She's taken it up, and golf galleries won't be the same after this. Before you protest that golf would seem a pedestrian choice for a star who does more moves than Deep Blue, IBM's chess-playing computer, may we speculate that she is venturing into this "rough" stuff to broaden her horizons and widen her outlook?

Certainly, if she ends up like any weekend hacker, she'll see—and hit—more wild blue yonder vistas than she ever thought possible: woods, farmers' fields, bunkers, and water. Lots and lots of water. Ponds, swimming pools, lakes, streams, rivers, and oceans. She'll learn that, unlike her dance style, where rules are what she makes of them, in golf there are boundaries that resound with out-of-bounds.

Shakira's proficient with the putter. After holing a 30 foot-plus putt, she shakes in exultation, a demonstration unlike any other golfer has ever given, not counting ex-basketball pro Charles Barclay's swing of strangeness.

Clearly Shakira's good on the greens. Jack Nicklaus was great on the greens, but does Shakira covet the crunched, hunched, and bunched putting pose of the Golden Bear in his later years? And what of Tiger? Can he focus on his faltering game or will his focus and foible come to the fore, should he ogle Shakira's form?

For the rest of us, this is not a moment of insouciance but an instance of celebration. If there is any sport that needs a jolt of energy (though Rory McIlroy, with his ups and downs, is doing his part) it's golf.

Anyway, Shakira has a full swing. Her follow-through is to die for. Her swing looks better than Arnold Palmer's ever did. She doesn't take the club back as far as "grip it and rip it" John Daly, but who does? The only problem is that the videographer, perhaps distracted by the young woman's fabulous faculties, zooms in on her, and we miss the golf balls' trajectories. Oh well.

This is swell—she teaches fundamentals: showing where best to set the ball for teeing off, laying her driver on the ground with the top end touching her left inside heel. (She's a righty, like most.) Unlike most ladies, save for Aussie Jan Stephenson on the women's tour years back, she has glamour, even wearing a plain white T-shirt, grey-sweat-pants ensemble.

When she talks of a straight left arm on the backswing and moving the hips— OK especially with moving the hips—she's eminently believable.

Where does she find the time? She tours—with her stellar singing career—all over the globe. She's into good causes as well, as founder of the Pies Descalzos Foundation, to assist Colombian children living in extreme poverty. Talking of the Hispanic community she said: "Not only do we represent the largest minority in the country, but the fastest growing; our community is in urgent need to provide all the necessary tools so that our children can develop their maximum potentials, talents, and intelligence."

Clearly, she's versatile. With this pretty darn good golf swing, she'll meet the sport's demands from tender-touch sand play to hacking the ball from heather. She'll master the deft chip and dominate the deep drive. Shakira seems at peace with herself (which is more than one can say for 99.9999% of weekend golfers and their games), putting her in good stead, as she steps ahead and brings her golf game to a climax.

Speaking of climax, where does it end? Shakira is certainly not the first superstar to take up golf but she may be the best at it. It speaks to the intricacies, idiosyncrasies, and impossibilities of golf that many otherwise talented people who try it can't play it, and can't even cope with it. Ex-basketball man Charles Barclay's swing will be analyzed by the kinesiologist and the sociologist years from now with a blustering: what the _ _ _ k!

Staying with the unreal for a moment, what is it with Colombia and delectable stars anyway? Surely Colombia's Camilo Villegas, declared the sexiest golfer on the tour in 2006 by *Golf Digest*, could fill the great guy-golfer bill. While he's wildly athletic (ever seen him read a putt?), there is room on the greens for the Barranquilla-born Shakira.

For ages, the PGA tour was a collective from the "University-of-Symmetry-in-similar-ball-flight-trajectory-with-all-sadly-singing-spin-from-the-same-19th-hole-interview-page-of-platitudes-in-homily." It was so boring, so snoring. It's now better with the aforesaid Rory—and with Ricky Fowler outfitted in the hot colors of the day—not that that's nearly the same as Shakira in any hue.

Thanks, however, to Shakira's rip-roaring thing with the golf swing, larger than life personas are once again okay in this sport and vice versa. Tiger Woods's philandering (no biggie there) and sourpussing(big bummer there) turned him into a tawdry spokesperson for the pastime. But now with the beautiful singer and dancer from Colombia picking up the niblicks specifically, and golf's pieces generally, once again the grand old game's future potential can spark some confidence and the hope of prosperity.

Unless she gyrates on to something new. No? Phew!

Chapter 30
Cross training—urban poling

You can use a pole to vault your way to cardio and core fitness. Don't think of the pole vault, however; think of pole walking, an activity adapted from Nordic walking.

The poles used are lightweight and height-adjustable, and are designed to help work upper body muscles. You can use them on trails or anywhere you fancy; they won't kill the budget and are easy to get the hang of. Indeed, a one-day, three to four-hour training course will have you on your way. Basically, the motions are the same as your standard walking stride, with the opposite arm and leg working in tandem as you step. You want to stand upright and keep your head up. For optimum results, keep the poles on an angle, more diagonal than vertical, allowing them to do what they do best: propel you forward.

So where and how does the core work come in? Get a grip. It's the slight pressure you put at the bottom of the pole handle that does the trick. That and keeping the abdominal muscles tight.

The only downside to pole walking is that it seems a bit dorky and nebbish. But if you end up taut and toned, who in their right mind is going to blather as much to your face? Let them talk behind your back; that's as it should be. And if they give you the gears and razz you as you pole on by, with your new strength you'll be able to whack 'em back.

Seriously, a study by the Cooper Institute in Dallas found that Nordic walking increased oxygen consumption, caloric expenditure, and heart rate significantly, without appreciably affecting the rate of exertion that the participants perceived.

Another plus is that the poles add stability to one's gait, which helps oldies or the injured get back on the path.

Chapter 31
Qigong and Tai Chi—Chinese medicine and martial arts

Qigong doesn't have it wrong. It has it bang on: "Stop. Breathe. Relax. " Three simple words, easy to understand. Three things to do, singly or in a group. That's not so simple.

Qigong is a blend of Chinese traditional medicine, philosophy, and martial arts. It's rooted in Taoism and Confucianism. It is not demanding drudgery like training for an ultra marathon, but it has prerequisites. The key is to be in the now, the moment, the present. Forget the past and forego the future as you go through the motions. Breathing and movement are not a forced synchronization; they harmonize naturally.

Described as medicine in motion, Qigong has been a godsend for arthritics. Adverse effects of Parkinson's, breast cancer, and insomnia have all been dimmed and dulled by Qigong, although researchers can't pinpoint what precise features of Qigong works on which particular facet(s) of these afflictions.

But they have some idea what the plusses are: increased blood flow to the brain; stress reduction; improved aerobic capacity; and a "striking immunity-boosting effect." (The latter finding was published in the *Journal of the American Geriatric Society*.)

Let me disclaim the heck out of everything here. Before doing Qigong or contemplating it as an option, adjunct, or alternative, consult your doctor. The "now hear this" out of the way, let's get back to our regular programming.

Qigong has been practiced for millennia in Asia. In the West, that fact has not been treated as a ringing endorsement. Acceptance of its purported benefits has been slow in coming. "Give me a rationale that fits with current Western medicine, or give me a break" has, quite often, been the reaction.

Most in the West have, however, heard of Tai Chi. It is a part of Qigong. Tai Chi is a Chinese martial art renowned for its sporting and health benefits. Research shows it helps with balance, a boon to seniors who take it up. Many pacifists wouldn't be caught dead in combat; they practice Tai Chi solely for its mental and physical benefits.

Nobody should embrace exercise without moderation, in harmony with one's own health situation. Qigong is all about that. Millions move to it but we must each incorporate it into our lifestyle individually.

Some dismiss Tai Chi as pedestrian, too slow and cerebral to stand up to other martial arts, like Karate for example. In this they would be wrong. Some forms of Tai Chi are formidable martial arts, worthy of respect from other martial arts disciplines. Don't let that slow, languid, "flowing like silk in the wind" appearance fool you. Watching a Qigong master move is like rubbing a kitten's fur between one's fingers: smooth, undulating, peaceful. Until the master strikes out—then you've got the cougar by the scruff.

Tai Chi, unlike so many other disciplines, does not have an international busy-body minding its P's and Q's. The advantage is avoidance of bureaucratic sclerosis; a disadvantage is that standards for instructors are nil, which enables some quacks to flourish unchallenged.

Can eighty million Chinese be mistaken? That is the estimated number of Chinese who practice Qigong daily. It puts individuals in charge of their own health care system, a far cry from the West where billions of dollars for health care goes down the drain while millions fatten up.

Qigong movement doesn't have to be snail-slow. There can be fast walking, turning, pivoting, and spinning motions, with pretty quick arm movements to boot, as Dr. Dharam Singh demonstrates on YouTube. It looks like the good doctor is having fun.

Clarity of spirit is a plus. Not sure what that means, but if one has the spirit to check this stuff out, maybe that's good enough for starters. For enders, well, there is no end. Qigong Master Chou was still spryly going through his paces at 92 (2008).

Qigong, with its self-massage, stances, movement, and breathing, has been a force in China for some 5,000 years. As early as 168 BC it was deemed a palliative for ailments like "…kidney disease, flatulence, painful knees, lumbago, rheumatism, gastric disturbance, and anxiety… "

Dementia is a demon that plagues some of us as we age. Exercise reduces the chances and effects of dementia but, for many older folks, a number of forms of exercise are too strenuous. This is where Tai Chi offers a great benefit. Because so many of the forms it takes are gentle, the elderly can shake a leg and shake off the shackles of senility in the process.

Qi, or Chi is the life force or energy flow. The literal meaning is air, breath, or gas. Qi is felt, built, stored, and circulated through meditative Qigong. The circulation of Chi can improve in as little as 10 minutes per day during which you breathe like a baby, through the belly, and not like an adult, through the chest.

A belly full of food hampers Qi circulation. Many of us pig out due to stress at home or work. Wouldn't it be a pleasant turnaround to use Qigong for a few minutes per day to not only lessen the strain but to lessen the weight?

Why wait?

Most of us, young or old, need a spark in our lives, emotionally, physically, and mentally. We crave stimulation. We want to catch the wave. Journey into Qigong and its Chi anytime, at any age; there are some *35,000 types of exercises* available.

We've all seen those folks in our parks, early in the morning, happily going about their business doing this stuff. It is contemplative and meditative, but it is physical conditioning as well. Trying to understand its many dimensions is like trying to catch flour falling through a sifter. Some parts, elusive, may never be caught, but one can always begin, try, and strive.

And be alive.

Chapter 32
Run along the 2012 Boston Marathon

(*Note:* The following was written before the horror of the 2013 bombings at the Boston Marathon. Let's hope that unspeakable terrorist tragedy does not deter marathoners from Boston, or other races.)

If you have to be a maniac and run a marathon, make it the Boston Marathon.

Why this marathon? It's the world's oldest annual marathon. It started back in 1897 and, if most of us lined up in that year, we'd just about be finished by now. 2012 is its 116th running.

Not enough for you? It's one of the five World Marathon Majors. Still not enough? You've been sloshing through sleet and stomping through snow non-stop (except for a nap here and there) six days out of the week in wild and wooly winter marathon torture training. Spring will come, officially at least, with the running of the Boston Marathon on April 16th, 2012. It's now time to take off those boots and put on those shoes.

Better make 'em jet propelled shoes. Because, according to sponsor John Hancock, these will be the fleetest men's and women's fields ever. Even last year's winners Caroline Kilel and Geoffrey Mutai, will be simultaneously sprinting, hopefully peaking, and peeking nervously over their shoulders to see who's coming on like gangbusters.

And Boston also has a gut wrencher in Heartbreak Hill. We'll collapse on that hill when we get to it momentarily.

You've got your special shoes. Now, if you're at least 18 years old on race day, okay, come on in. But only if you have met qualifying race speed standards as set out by the Boston Athletic Association (B.A.A.) The timings are age appropriate, not that it's appropriate for anyone, at any age, to run 26 miles and 385 yards.

Just to give you an idea of how fast you gotta be, consider: for men 18 to 34—3 hours 10 minutes; for women—3 hours 40 minutes. Call it a mixed gender bag of 3 hours 25 minutes. That works out to roughly 7.88 minutes per mile. This is faster than an 8 minute mile—which is a run, not a jog.

If you are a geezer, take a breather. If 80+ and a man, your 5 hours time should do the trick. For the geezerette, a 5 hour, 30 minute pace will see you in the race.

And all wannabe runners—get into this year's race because apparently the 2013 qualifying standards will be even tougher—by 5 minutes!

And if you are blind or in a wheelchair, or can't ambulate properly, you get a break too. Of course the biggest, smartest break would be to stay home. Which leads us to the question: Why do people run marathons?

No sane person knows why. There were 26,895 runners in the 2011 Boston Marathon who await diagnosis. Let's move on…

Can Geoffrey Mutai beat his 2:03:02 time set in the Boston Marathon 2011? He and other speedsters in that 115th edition (2011) had, besides super stamina and fantastic form, the aid of tailwinds. But even the beneficence of Mother Nature cannot diminish the significance of any racer who actually finishes.

For first timers, there is a clinic on March 26th, 2012, that tells you basically how to stay on route, including a course preview with dietary recommendations (like don't eat 12 hot dogs before the race) and a session that speaks to proper clothing (how not to wear your pumps and parka). After that, you are all set.

Geez, even a quick glance at the Boston Marathon 2012 route gives you the willies. There is, of course, the aforementioned Heartbreak Hill. But from start to finish, from the bottom left to the top right on the map, it gives the impression of being all uphill. That can't be true, can it? (No.)

What is certainly true is the amalgam of objects and humanity on Heartbreak Hill: cheering, clapping, hooting spectators, officials on motorcycles, official trucks and cars, and, here and there, even some participants. Mutai was so blazing fast in 2011 as to resemble a Tour de France cyclist, although he runs clean.

And it *is not* the sheer displacement of Heartbreak Hill that causes shudders and mental-physical lock up, it's the Hill's sinister position in the race. Although only (only?!) an 88 foot vertical ascent over .40 of a mile, the spirit-squashing, soul-destroying abomination occurs between the 20th and 21st miles. By this time most runners' energy is sapped; they're running on fumes. And to meet and beat this…

… takes a special kind of nut.

Competitors run differently. They'll have varied racing time differentials. But no matter who you are, during training, rest and recuperation are critical to arriving at Hopkinton (the start) *not* in a broken down heap. Whether it's one day off a week or every two weeks—without that time away from training, mentally and physically, a personal best is likely *not* in the offing. And don't leave the "starting blocks" pistons pumping. Save some strength for the second half, including Heartbreak Hill.

Remember this too: "the B.A.A. does not assume responsibility for runners' health, safety, security, or support… "

And the weather can vary as much as the mood in a séance. In 2004 it was a sizzling 83 degrees. In 2007 it was a chilly 47.

Finish up with a foaming beer. Just don't offer to buy a round, otherwise the approximately half a million roadside fans might belly up to your billfold. For this 2012 Boston Marathon, a new beer will be on tap: Adams Boston 26.2 Brew. In sync with the race premise of health and heartiness, it is a light beer.

To run the Boston Marathon is a testament to dedication, diligence, and determination. To finish is a result of superior training and eating. To talk of your exploits to friends and family is to be expected, accepted, and enjoyed. To do the whole thing again?

Is loopy—and living!

Note: Mutai had to drop out without finishing in 2012, though other Kenyan runners finished in first, second, and third place in both the men's and women's divisions.

Chapter 33
Does the NFL stand for the National Fat League?

And now for some surprising struggles of pro athletes...

You've wowed family and friends, wooed your prospective agent, worshiped your coach, survived grueling training camps, abided punishing practices, coped with four-day physical and mental interrogations at the NFL Scouting Combine, tolerated pumping iron, dealt with bone-crushing tackles and mind-numbing blocking assignments, and finally, memorized mesmerizing offensive plays and learned backwards and forwards byzantine defensive forays. You've done all of this, and more—only to be classified by some pointy-headed academics as obese? That's a chop block, a hit below the belt, a cheap shot if there ever was one.

So what's the score? It's true.

Lo! Beware the leviathan, the loadstone, the humungous hump of humanity. And watch how that beast broadly fills your wide-screen TV. That's what one solitary lineman of the NFL is corpulently capable of.

When push comes to shove, call it two pounds per year. Or up to that. Since 1942 linemen have gained .7 to two pounds per year. By the year 2050 we could have 400-plus pound defensive ends. Break the barrel of dip and deliver to me the crate of chips! Should we par*tay*?

Sure. Why not? We aren't the ones who will have to carry that weight around for the rest of our lives until the gridiron's grim reaper calls an audible at the line of fatality. Once defensive linemen, in their endless pursuit of quarterbacks and once offensive tackles in relentless protection of those same quarterbacks are retired, so much of that muscle might, with easy living, ebb. And so much blubber might, with a more sedentary lifestyle, flow. And we observers won't be beset and upset, as they will be, with metabolic disorders, the depression that comes of no longer garnering publicity, the downer of having no fans, and the disappearance of the entourage from the heady days of a pro ball career.

Here's an entourage of a different sort. Call it a wrap around 11%.

That's the average body fat percentage gained since 1942. Does this fact bother coaches? Not at all. In fact, many coaches drool at getting the next Aaron Gibson. Who dat, you say? Before he retired in 2004, after playing a total of 38 games over six years, Aaron was thought to be the biggest bloke on the NFL block, smothering the scale at 440 pounds. A look at his profile on Pro-Football-Reference.com has his weight at 375 pounds. A possible yo-yo weight problem?

You tell him that.

But we've got coaches who won't tell him that his weight could be a problem for him later. They are all hot and bothered about the next big body beautiful. And we've got youngsters who surely won't even wonder. They are too busy huffing and puffing, salivating and hyperventilating, and perhaps toying with steroids, looking to fill those big-body-beautiful pads with their pie-in-the-sky pro football dreams—and the combination of accentuated training and exaggerated feeding has produced some startling results.

Consider the Panthers of Elder High School in Ohio. The football team is not in the neighborhood of sleek, nor in the solar system of meek, they're in the fifth dimension of eek! with 10 players that weigh over 250 pounds.

On their official Web site, the coaches talk of helping the boys grow "…not only intellectually but also physically, spiritually, culturally and socially." They certainly have the "physically" aspect down pat. Talk about your gravy train.

The thickening of the players has been shouted out loud since at least 2005. Back then, a study found that 56% of NFL players could be considered obese.

And as the Associated Press reported, those coaches who worshiped at the altar of mammoth, should have then, and perhaps now, taken notes: In the 2003–2004 season, Arizona players lumbered in, BMI-wise, as the biggest. But they weren't the best. Far from it. In fact, the fatties were slack, racking up the lousiest record in their division.

Many are shooting the messenger—the BMI or Body Mass Index—claiming that it is misleading in that it does not account for body muscle, as opposed to fat. Detractors also claim that the study, led by endocrinologist Dr. Joyce Harp, was faulty because data from the NFL website for 2,168 players for the 2003–2004 season could be skewed—giant actual weights were reported as Goliath non-factual weights. Teams, it was suggested, aren't above intimidation by any means possible in their desire to mess with their opponents' heads.

Here's a bit of a headscratcher. The NFL proudly promotes its fitness campaign. But it's for kids. Started in 2007, Play 60 encourages kids to hack around (physically, not on the computer) for at least an hour a day. The encouragement is backed by dough ($200 million and counting), advertisements, and initiatives partnered in the 32 cities where the teams are based.

But if the child grows up to be a defensive lineman, according to a study by the National Institute of Occupational Safety and Health sent to NFL retirees in 2012, heart disease could be a game breaker. It has led to membership in the

Six-Feet-Under Club for these behemoths in greater numbers than for the average guy, final score: 41 deaths versus the expected 29.

One ex-Pro Bowl guard, Keith Sims, is increasing awareness among other huge, retired players about the perils of obesity. And Sims leads by example. He has had lap-band surgery. He is a spokesman for the NFL Retired Players Heart Obesity Prevention Education and Referral Program that will conduct physicals on retired players to tell them what's what with their waists, width, and whatnot. The ardent hope is that retired players will listen to one of their own, and will feel more pre-disposed to voice their concerns, questions, and comments. Sims can offer ready alternatives, if not outright answers.

The NFL is not in a hurry to discuss this issue. Its Fall 2012 Health and Safety Report discusses women's breast cancer, reports on men's prostate cancer, expounds on child obesity, informs about traumatic brain injury, pontificates on clean competition (anti-doping), reflects on staph infections, deliberates on dementia, and then finally, on page 24 of 29, gets around to outlining how its Cardiovascular Health Subcommittee is on the case of player obesity.

As much as it's a valid concern, the plight of the active or retired NFL player saddled with obesity is nothing compared to that of the amateur high school player who won't make pro. The kids have no support groups, like the one Keith Sims speaks for above, or the NFL Player Care Foundation (NFLPA) to help them sort out issues when their sporting days are over. And what about the injuries suffered by smaller high school players after colliding with their obese opponents? Those statistics can't be pretty.

But let's get back to basics for a moment and deal with the case of the BMI. Is it getting a bum rap? Or is it worth its weight in calories in calculating obesity?

Consider, if you will, the case of hockey superstar Sidney Crosby...

Chapter 34
Sidney Crosby Hexed by body mass index?

Back in March of 2011 folks were wondering…

Is Sidney Crosby hexed by the Body Mass Index (BMI)? Is the BMI a pie in the sky, an irrelevant yardstick for obesity? Is it on its way to oblivion? And should it be? Why? Consider Canadian hockey superstar Sidney Crosby who plays for the Pittsburgh Penguins. Apparently Crosby has a high BMI rating. He's a tub of lard in Penguin hockey gear. Oh dear.

What is the BMI? It is a formula. BMI = weight in pounds/(height in inches × height in inches) × 703. *The 703 is to convert the index from the original metric system used to create the formula* to the Imperial system (pounds and ounces).

Let's see how this works: You are 5'4". In cm that equals approx. 162.5; take that plus your weight of 148 pounds and see where they intersect on the graph.

You will be in the C Zone which reads "may lead to health problems." Just yesterday, for the first time in your life, you bench pressed more than your weight and are the strongest you have ever been. The only health problem you are aware of is a zest and pang for more of this same health. The BMI, in arbitrarily smashing weight against height, can be worse than useless, it is misleading.

And as for Sidney Crosby, though his earnings may help offset the slings and arrows of outrageous typecasting by some BMI dimwit twit, he's now stigmatized. So, on the bright side, he's a victim, with all the societal booty and benefit such a branding incurs.

So the BMI is thin if it is used a means to calculate fatness. Don't believe what you read and see here? Check out the Health Canada BMI Nomogram. What the heck is a Nomogram? It is a fancy way of saying chart. But what is not so fancy is how Health Canada, after touting the BMI's merits, disclaims the whole deal with "qualifiers," "what ifs," and "on the other hands" to mean that one should take many factors that may impact body weight and health into consideration. Factor them in, fudge them out, then and only then may you treat the BMI as a half-assed indicator of something or other.

Back in July 2009, a mathematician and senior researcher at Stanford University Keith Devlin, came up with 10 reasons as to why the BMI is, in his words, bogus.

Hey hey, ho ho, the BMI has got to go, give it a throw. Don't despair about that weight as measured by BMI. That way of thinking is so March 9th, 2011. In a 2011 study in the medical journal *Lancet*, researchers said, in more unified and louder voices than ever before, that the BMI—which does not separate or differentiate between muscle and fat when summing body weight—isn't a good indicator of weight, obesity, and perceived associated problems. They say, don't waste time with the BMI, spend time focusing on the waist, the circumference of the body where the waist makes the body go round. Crucial, this.

Not surprisingly these new voices haven't convinced everyone. Dr. Ali Zentner, a specialist in internal medicine, feels that people whose BMI is over 30 are obese. Period. She does qualify that, however, saying that the BMI is but a first step in diagnosis. Moreover, she feels BMI could use an ethnocultural tweak.

So what does "ethnocultural" mean? It refers to the fact that people of Chinese, Cuban, Scottish, or Aboriginal origin, to cite a few examples, have different patterns of behavior and their diet choices will naturally influence their body weights and health. How does that affect obesity and BMI? We can rank obesity by country, and those countries with a predominant ethnocultural group may shed light on obesity statistics in a multi-ethnic nation such as the United States or Canada. The USA ranks 5th amongst the top 10 countries in the world for obesity, as of 2008. The United Kingdom ranks 9th and New Zealand 10th. Quite possibly, the UK, like the USA, is more multicultural than New Zealand or number one, Cook Islands, or number two, Tonga.

(This just in. Mexico, as of 2013, is now deemed the most obese country in the developed world, surpassing the USA. So says a new United Nations report.)

Three factors are used to measure obesity: the BMI, the waist circumference calculation, and the co-morbid risks—diabetes, arthritis, heart disease, etc., that are more common among obese persons. Right now the jury is still out on whether the circumference calculation will do the job any better than the, perhaps discredited, BMI does. Check out this startling news from March 11th, 2011, headlined "Weight Measure May Not Be Major Predictor of Heart Disease." Reading through the article it was tough to tell, what with all the jargon what the latest Cambridge study found. It found that the Waist Circumference Inference wasn't all it was cracked up to be either.

So leaving co-morbid risks out of the loop, what are we left with to accurately assess obesity? Maybe we'll have to summon our innermost feelings to decide if we, or others in the sauna, are obese, given that the medical and scientific world keeps throwing their hands in the air over new studies that negate or lessen earlier ones. Or maybe we'll have to feel each other up. Do you feel obese? I think you feel great. Maybe that will have to do, until the next BMI or obesity paper hits the journals.

Chapter 35
Land sakes! Golfer John Daly hits 6 in lake!

Other than Tiger Woods and Rory McIlroy, is there any golfer more fun to watch than "Wild Thing" John Daly? It's not just the "grip it and rip it" mentality that so enraptures crowds, it's that you don't know whether he or the ball will get teed off first.

Let's hope big John (although he has slimmed down some) doesn't become a spectacle just for being a crazy coot. The guy has—had—an amazing touch around the greens for a fellow who could swat the ball a country mile and win two majors. Some might argue (unsuccessfully, most would agree) that winning one major is a fluke—anybody can fool 'em for four rounds in four days—but to win two, with one being the historic British Open—well, that's no freak of nature.

Betcha you didn't know that Mr. Daly was the fourth American since World War II to win two majors before his 30th birthday. Jack Nicklaus, Tom Watson, and Johnny Miller were the others

In recent years, John has had more trouble on the golf course than he's had with wives (he has had four wives). But with that everyman look, and common man frailty—he still garners interest and appeal no matter where he goes. People would *love* to see him make it back, to finish high in a tournament. Winning one more would give him worldwide headlines.

So what's John done recently to make the media happy and the purists grumpy? He seems to have gone over the top in the Land Down Under. In the Australian Open *he hit 6 shots into a lake*. We hackers can relate. He quit after the 11th hole at The Lakes Golf Club. How many of us have thrown our clubs en masse into the nearest body of water or flung at least one down the fairway? Or snapped several irons over our knee?

The problem, of course, is that a national golf tournament carries with it a country's prestige. The onus is on the player to be respectful of the host's hospitality, to praise the course condition and volunteers as needed, and compliment both no matter what. People are watching. Closely.

The Aussies are none too pleased: Championship director Trevor Herden cited Daly for unprofessional conduct. Others say John Daly has no balls. A YouTube video, online in the summer of 2013, shows his last shot plunking into a lake.

Should he have sucked it up and continued playing, knowing full well he wouldn't be making the cut and would waste the next round and that day? Probably. Sometimes work does seem useless but one must trudge on, regardless.

Sure, he self-destructed in a wet-ball-shower of self-immolation but hey, the 11th hole was a dog leg par 5, a 528 meter beast, with a lurking lake. It would have been worse, but not out of the realm of possibility and more fun still, had Daly found water on another hole he wasn't currently playing and unceremoniously sank a few in there.

As snits go, this wasn't a great one. He didn't storm off so much as walk off. He shook hands with somebody. His caddy couldn't have been too pleased, but if you opt to carry the bags for long John Daly, you know the pitfalls going in.

And it is hardly unheard of. No less than Tiger Woods has had some power pouts. But if John can't pattern himself after the young shot makers of today he could go "extreme sport," reach into his old bag of tricks, and whip out some tantrum imitations of yore. Tommy Armour comes to mind.

Let's get it straight from the horse's mouth—or at least from John Daly's Twitter feed—on the 11th hole doings and dunkings:

> when u run out of balls u run out of balls. yes, I shook my player's
> partners hands & signed my card w/rules official.

It may be official but it borders on lackadaisical, farcical. How many balls are allowed in a round of tournament play? Of course, no one in their right mind, or with the right shots, could envision leaving six in the lake, but you'd think that to fly all that way to only have to forfeit because you had no balls…

Herden says Daly's not welcome back at the Australian Open. He is frustrated that he can't fine Daly. Herden hoped, however, that the US and European Tour officials find the fortitude to reprimand John or maybe re-seed him six feet under. Just kidding on that last point. But the sentiment is there.

With four wives, drinking dilemmas, drug accusations, dietary demons, and a love of all things Razorback, John Daly's "larger than life" life is more colorful than New Year's Eve fireworks put on by a mad team of Mardi Gras exhibitionists. "Stuff" like his travails in the Australian Open are, ahem, par for the course.

His fourth marriage to Sherrie Miller was a disastrous doozie, so maybe that vexing temptation many of us succumb to—of putting the possibility of hope over the sad-but-true reality of eternal, infernal marriages—is behind him now. He put his weight problems to rest with Lap-Band surgery. Oh, if only it were that easy to solve one's golf or personal predicaments by walking into a clinic and coming out copasetic! But it *is* for all his warts and wanton ways that John Daly remains an edgy icon to this day. He epitomizes the tons of dark troubles and tidbits of bright triumphs that most of us experience.

Chapter 36

Pursuing excellence, modeled by Tiger Woods

If it's good enough for Tiger Woods, it should be good enough for you and me. What's good enough for Tiger Woods? That he isn't good enough. Before you think this is silly circular logic, do you remember his story? Tiger Woods, already the best golfer of his time and recognized by many in the know as possibly the best golfer of all time, is constantly looking to improve, still hungry to get better.

Admirable.

Even though he's driven, no pun intended, far more than most of us, that doesn't mean we shouldn't learn from this Tiger beast. Just as he decided he could learn from Hank Haney. Despite world-shattering success with prior golf swing coach Butch Harmon, Tiger, in his relentless pursuit of excellence, decided to switch coaches. That was, in and of itself, a huge move, and it entailed an overhaul of Tiger's swing. Now the golf world may argue the specific merits of Tiger's penchant for switching coaches and altering his swing but…

Okay, here we must come to a full stop. In no way would a sane person recommend you overhaul your weightlifting techniques, for example, if they are generally sound. But you should grasp the gist of what Tiger's doing and pursue the same ongoing quest to better yourself, to learn the whys and wherefores of what you do. Negate complacency. Perfection may be impossible but near perfection should be in your golf bag. Aim high, and see what kind of "scores" you reap.

Beep, beep, this just in. In 2010 Tiger Woods yet again reviewed his game and picked up Sean Foley as his swing coach. Tiger, having won the Arnold Palmer Invitational in March 2013, vaulted back as the world's top golfer, the ranking he had last held 125 weeks earlier. And Tiger, being no fool, didn't pick a slouch of a teacher. Sean Foley's work with Justin Rose has been admirable, taking Rose from number 76 in the world to number 5.

The point is that all of us, just like Tiger, should persevere in our pursuit of the possible, and perch as near as possible to perfection.

Chapter 37
Aerial silks exercise exudes grace and guts

A little bit off the beaten track, but...

Aerial silks exercise is the latest craze in fitness. With a difference. It frees your imagination to picture yourself a Lara Croft, releasing the body to perform upside down and all around undulations and permutations that one would never have thought possible.

Aerial silk is a piece of cloth with its center suspended from above. Dare-devil participants say it elevates, enervates, titillates. And irritates: Swollen knuckles and calluses are common, at least initially. To the sedentary watcher, it is a spacey, surreal vista—an angelic soar above the floor—made for body bends and contortions.

And moving through thin air forces the aerialist to focus on body form and function. Exercises can't be sloughed off haphazardly.

Aerial silks is not aerial yoga. The latter involves yoga moves in mid-air while the former consists of a fluid, suspended dance of climbs, drops, and poses. Women fill the majority of aerial silks classes.

Aerial silks demands diligence and thought. When one is suspended upside down, babbling to a buddy about how school or work is going doesn't come naturally.

The "silk" is usually polyester. Silk sounds sweet. It has a certain cachet. But polyester is utilitarian and offers varying flexibilities. And anyone trying this exercise had better have good elbow and knee joints because they will take a considerable amount of strain. Also, if you are quite overweight, stick to ground training before you attempt this. But aerial silks is certainly something to shoot for, if only to try it once.

And careful with the groin; don't swan off into your version of the Russian splits—otherwise it may take much more than Humpty Dumpty's men to put you back together again.

Most of us haven't done anything kinda crazy since our days on the monkey bars. How fun it would be to turn back time and just act goofy, inwardly at least, as we swing very carefully into shape.

Watching acrobatic aerialists breeze through the air many feet above the ground—and safety—is to watch apparent effortlessness—even though we know that their routines take extreme effort and are most definitely not a breeze.

For the newcomer, it may be all you can do to not strangle yourself, ensnarled in the fabric. Coming out alive, with all body parts *not* drawn and quartered, might be considered a worthy accomplishment.

And don't worry too much about a long fall, for in beginners' aerial silks classes, the distance from the base of the fabric to the floor can be easily touched by either toe or finger, depending on which digit is closest at that time.

Let's say you have decided to try flapping, fumbling, and floundering with this regimen. Your upper body strength will be formidably taxed. Just tell everybody that you are trying to get the hang of: Aerial Tissue, Flying Silks, Aerial Curtain, Aerial Fabric, Aerial Chiffon, and Aerial Dance. It will sound *much more* complex and complicated, and you'll be cut some slack.

But there is no slack with this air athletics program. Watching the spine arc backwards is unnerving. But gazing at arms and hands and legs and feet extended for a purpose is beautiful, like aerial repose enwrapped in pantyhose…

Whether you are dealing with basic movements for the legs or for the arms, just viewing the process makes it crystal clear that the arm strength needed to climb up the strand is critical, as is core and abdomen strength to keep your body in a tight pose as you lower or extend your legs away from a vertical to a horizontal position.

This might sound crazy but it reminds me of swimming. How so? The two sports both have a "dear life" factor. With aerial silks you have to hold on for dear life; otherwise you could, even from a short distance, give your head a nasty crack on a fall. With swimming, if you don't swim for dear life, you'll drown.

And beginners, whatever you do—do not ever work out with aerial silks without an instructor or coach. And check to see whose insurance covers this caper, yours or the club's.

One basic essential move, to prevent the splat-drat fall, is the footlock. The fabric is enwrapped around one or two feet, so if you lose your grip you at least have contact, no matter how tenuous, with the ribbon through that foot-fold hold.

And extending your legs out in a jackknife, well, the quadriceps muscles will seem like a quivering fire. The hamstrings, too, look to be stretched to their limits. Unlike a slow stretch on the ground where pace, rate, and distance is controlled, with aerial silks it looks much harder to prevent your legs (or arms) from stretching, or elongating, much faster than intended.

The aerial hammock looks like a much safer bet for a chicken like myself—and even that looks like a swing too far because you do let the body "go"—or at least the professional or accomplished acrobat types do. If you were scuba diving, you'd have water filling every gap where your body isn't, as you maneuver. You'd have support. But with aerial silks, the support comes from thin threads: the fabric itself, your body strength, and your sense of body awareness, balance, and athleticism.

It's fun to watch. That's as far as I'll go myself. Except to say that my respect for this discipline has risen with observation, and my heart rate, watching and learning about aerial silks, has shot up higher still.

Chapter 38
Drumstick-smashing pound class workout

Get fit with drumsticks and rap-tap-tap the fat back at Pound Class? What? With Pound (whacking drumsticks), you will *know* you are part of the latest Hollywood fitness fad-and-fave to hit the gyms.

For years, music has provided a backdrop to fitness classes. A brainwave that two cerebral, highly conditioned women had at a party sparked a collision in collusion.

The blend became known as "drumstick-smashing." It is not to be confused with the kettlebell workout we will look at next, which took over Hollywood fitness, as did drumstick-smashing. Both are fads that may last. Drumstick's creators, Cristina Peerenboom and Kirsten Potenza, say that smashing is fun, mixes Pilates with drumming, and leaves one feeling like a rock star. Their fitness routines were inspired by ex-Guns N' Roses drummer, Matt Sorum.

Technically, you don't need a gym. But, to trip out, you do need weighted drumsticks called Ripstix, a love of raising Cain, and some understanding neighbors. Then you too can lower that body weight, via this resistance training, on any old floor in your home. But use rubber mats.

Drumming to a throbbing beat... like in the musical *Stomp*—who knows how low that weight can go? The drumsticks are a delightful distraction: you're not focused on the rigors of lunges, squats, or core work, with drumsticks to hand.

Essentially the Ripstix are light hand weights. They are plastic, weighing one pound each. What a blast, working that whole body while releasing pent-up, pug-ugly tension and frustration in the process. You can see—*and hear*—the results, gauge how your rhythm's coming along, and ascertain whether you are "at one" with others in the class.

Let's say you are having trouble keeping up, that you drum with the proverbial two left feet. Not to worry. The idea is not to prove you are the second coming of Billy Cobham, though that'd be a bonus. It *is* to boost that cardio strength and blow out—how many calories per session? It's been described as a Trojan Horse, sneaking in a chance to burn up 700–900 calories.

The POUND-Rockout Workout is inexpensive; drumsticks and an instructional DVD cost nowhere near the range of a Stair Climber, some weird strap contraption, or a Nautilus set.

Getting this new fitness program to become commercially viable was not easy. Kirsten Potenza, ex-UCLA coxswain rower and sociology major, and Cristina Peerenboom, class of 2008 neuroscience at the University of Arizona and fitness instructor, needed independent financing to get their boat afloat.

Both founders played drums in high school. We all remember our buddies playing those drums—standing up—in our teen years. With Pound, a full range of body motion, geared to specially designed choreographic sequences, has the participant beating the sticks standing on both feet, on one foot, lying on the stomach or the back, flailing them rapid-fire. This "Pilates with drumming" is humming. One can reach 160 beats per minute this way, good for cardio and good for sweat.

Classes run for 45 minutes. After-class stiffness can last for hours, but to an aching man and woman, newcomers enthuse about and muse on the workout's merits. Another great thing about Pound? Just that, Pound. Don't look for euphemisms here. Pound means pound, no pussy-footing around.

So, yes, drumstick-smashing is the new winsome workout favorite. Does it have something many fitness choices don't? With most fitness programs, you've got two things going for you: looking good and feeling good—two out of three ain't bad. But what about a Trifecta? How marvy would it be to look way cooler than you used to? With Pound, you are going to look *way cooler* than you would with urban pole walking. Hands down. No contest.

What's also incontestable and incontrovertible is the thwack attack's effect on one's demeanor. Unleashing demons with Pound, without the so played-and-staid passé primal screams, is a step up, a social good. Take a tantrum to task, slapping and whapping those rubber mats histrionically.

Currently, let's kill two birds with one stone, why don't we? Gotta bend down in our cardio-stretching disciplines anyway: isn't it *way more* of a toot to tap-tap-tap those sticks instead of mindlessly touching those tippy toes?

No doubt, as the beat goes on, a new fun fitness regimen will push Pound to the sidelines somewhat, and that's fine. That's the nature of the fitness biz, and that's life. But right now Pound, along with getting great press reaction from no less than the *New York Times, The Doctors,* and the *Los Angeles Times,* is getting around in corporate wellness programs, Pilates studios, dance studios, and Crunch gyms. And like gadgets, for sure your first set of drumsticks will get a flurry of novelty use. But unlike gadgets, they'll surely maintain their utility and popularity and *won't get* relegated to the attic, only to be brought out as an afterthought when the grandkids come by.

Fun should be part and parcel of all our lives, and fitness should be a bag we carry always and everywhere. Drumstick smashing seems to cover both those bases.

Kirsten and Cristina seem to have covered all the bases too. Kirsten's philosophy of life, if favorite quotes from her Facebook page are any indication, is: Life is not a dress rehearsal. That's smashing, even without the drumsticks. Pound that.

Chapter 39

Adore Thor, for Chris Hemsworth is swell with the kettlebell

Thor, the blockbuster action flick, has raked in mega-millions, and its blond, tousled-haired lead Chris Hemsworth is more than just a pretty face. The Australian is a pretty near perfect, rock-hard hero of Herculean proportions himself. How did he land the starring role in this gravy train of a hit movie?

Well, he made his mettle from metal, specifically from the iron kettlebell. Chris, according to his trainer Mike Knight, used a 44-pounder for his "Triple Crush" exercises, with lots of oomphs undoubtedly thrown in.

How long have kettlebells been around? They were first used in markets as a counterweight in Mother Russia as far back as the 1700s. The Russians swept the throwing events in the 1980 Olympics due to kettlebell training. Actor Gerard Butler, in preparation for his role as King Leonidas in the flick *300*, used them. You and I can go bad-ass ballistic with one. Literally. The "cannon ball with a handle" is meant for ballistics exercises. What are ballistics exercises? Throwing explosive ones, like those used in bench throws and jump squats. The Greek word, *ballein*, is the basis for ballistic.

Why are we all agog over demigod Chris Hemsworth in *Thor*? Because his ardent, assiduous training has honed his fast-twitch muscle fibers to seemingly hyper speeds: he heaves that hammer and we breathe in adulation.

Certainly Thor, and anyone who undertakes such body-taxing exertions, earns an ovation. Here's what's involved, and what is at risk if the exercise is not done properly. Don't start out catapulting the kettlebell straight away—for sure you'll get all screwed up and blow a gasket. If you've a bad back, soft shoulders, or a cushy core—don't go near the kettlebell, other than to gawk at it. Otherwise it's the kettlebell from Hell.

But if you slowly build up training, through weights, with exercises carefully applied to affect all the necessary body parts, then the American Council on Exercise says, for starters, that a 15–25 pound kettlebell may be for the man in you. And the ultimate reward is the Valhalla of a bodacious body as heavenly as Chris Hemsworth's.

And what of Thor's thunderous throw? In the Prose Edda of Norse mythology, we are told that Thor: "... would be able to strike as firmly as he wanted, whatever his aim, and the hammer would never fail, and if he threw it at something, it would never miss and never fly so far from his hand that it would not find its way back, and when he wanted, it would be so small that it could be carried inside his tunic." Carry this tip everywhere.

Michigan-based fitness trainer to the stars, Mike Knight, comes from a position of strength, specifically the Art of Strength (AOS). Mike is one of 64 certified Art of Strength kettlebell instructors in the United States. He tells the story of a man—himself—whose shoes we would not want to walk in.

Why? Because he was 100 pounds overweight, a couple of years away from death according to his doctor, and had to lose all that weight the hard, no-shortcut way, through training and proper diet. Nobody in their right mind needs to balloon up to a beach ball before Mike's lessons are learned. One of his major breakthroughs has been with the kettlebell. Used properly, the kettlebell can *reduce* the chance of injury.

The NHL's Detroit Red Wings, super for years on end, and the NFL's Detroit Lions, usually stinky for decades to never end, both swear and sweat by Mike Knight's regimen which involves, along with the kettlebell, taking sledge hammers to huge tires, side-to-side jumping, huge barbell-weighted curls and rope exercises that kind of look like skipping.

As of May 16th, there were 119 million reasons to train with a kettlebell, if the worldwide box office gate for *Thor* is any indication. And perhaps some of that money will be quickly spent on deluxe high-end trainers—for they are not cheap, $300 per hourly session being ballpark.

We don't want a level playing field. We want the edge. What is the verdict on training with weights and/or the kettlebell? The jury is in, having made its decision, and both of the latter are winners; the only remaining question is the degree and type of effort. Put simply, the more you put in safely, the more you'll get out successfully.

What man wouldn't give his right arm (nope that doesn't sound quite right, maybe not *that* much) to look as out-of-this-world as Chris Hemsworth does? Maybe getting that maestro-marvel of a fitness trainer might be the best money he ever spent.

Thor might be in a bit of trouble, a bit spent these days, for the 4th Pirates of the Caribbean movie, *On Stranger Tides* is a serious competitor in the genre. But that's no excuse for us to shy, shirk, and shrink away from strength exercises. Heed and obey. Ascend from hapless and helpless to hardy and hale, and like Chris Hemsworth's Thor, throw caution to the wind, fling that hammer, toss off that T-shirt, and be a killer whale with your great tale, and tail.

Chapter 40
Senior citizens and body-building

Grandpas and Grandmas are tightening up and getting skimpy in swim suits. Their outlooks now are as large as their body fat percentages are small, and a sweet sixteen of them are strutting and pumping their stuff.

Back around 2008, for example, we learned that in the five years, "the number of men and women in their sixties and seventies competing in United States Body-building Federation shows has doubled to 16," according to Brian Washington, the commissioner of the federation, a drug-free group.

Ah yes, the drugs, or rather the freedom therefrom. Are these seniors showing off on stage sans steroids? Well, the USBF home page touts "Natural Athletes" and "fair and objective drug testing" as a priority. Some seniors probably do take supplements, but they generally abhor steroids and human growth hormones.

For these select sixteen or so older folks, the trend is a happy one. They are raising the bar of the body beautiful while lowering their non-chronological ages to the lowest levels possible through body-building. If this trend catches on, it might put more than a few plastic body-repair surgeons on the bread line.

And then there is Sir Charles Eugster.

A chin-up is almost impossible to do. Sixty-one chin-ups in 45 seconds are unthinkable. That a 91-year-old man could muscle up that feat is unfathomable. And fantastic. And drastic. Yet Sir Charles Eugster can do it! He's the 91-year-old body-builder, who didn't burst into these brawny he-man heroics until he was in his late eighties.

It's never too late to say "now or never."

Most of us get in shape, lose it, then get it back again. Sadly, for so many of us, there is a last time after which we never get it back.

It was almost like that for Eugster. He looked into the mirror, searched his soul, and starkly realized that his life, while not over at 85, was a sad sack excuse for what he wanted to be, and see.

Now he's checking and charting in with chin-ups, dips, push-ups, and crunches. In bunches. How about us?

Few of us are centenarians, folks who live past the age of 100. Those who do exhibit some common characteristics, as itemized in John W. Santrock's book, *A Topical Approach to Life-Span Development*. These characteristics include five factors that research has suggested are crucial to longevity 1) heredity and family history 2) health, i.e. weight, diet, whether or not a person smokes, amount of exercise 3) education level 4) personality 5) lifestyle.

Back to body-building, or weight training. Would it benefit seniors to, ahem, pick this activity up? Well, that depends. If flexibility is added to a weight training program, then it might be a good idea. But if flexibility and a stretching regimen are not practiced simultaneously, then you might have a gristly-gnarled geezer ready to tip.

Regimen this, senior citizens of America. Do something. Do anything. After consulting your doctor, of course. Forty percent of women and 30% of men over 70 admit that they do no exercise in their daily lives.

Why wait for weights, flexibility, and cardio? Reverse aging by 15 years via a 45-minute workout daily. Watch strength increase 75 to 100%. Know that bone density is increasing by 1 to 2%. All possible, according to Miriam Nelson, an associate professor of nutrition at Tufts University.

Not only can senior shapes spring back from sedentary sloth, senior brains will sharpen, perhaps stemming the scourge of dementia. Vonda Wright, an expert on exercise and aging at the University of Pittsburgh Medical Center, advises that exercise also produces a neuron growth factor that stimulates the brain. That may be the reason it apparently protects against memory loss and alleviates depression.

With flexibility, cardio, and weights as the watchwords and ways three, arthritis can abate and fractures, cruelly common to seniors, can be greatly reduced or prevented as well.

Did you know that there is an International Council on Active Aging? Their site's Consumer section is chock full of useful "stuff" for seniors to peruse and use.

Just remember, and this goes not only for seniors, but for most of us: Don't go too far, too fast, or else injury may invite itself in. Up those weights in training by 1- to 2-pound (.45 – to .91 kg) increments. Some elder-friendly gyms offer these more graduated levels. More are getting them. All need them.

Let's take a break and get the take on aging from some wits, wags, thinkers, and celebrities.

Bette Davis: "Growing old is not for sissies."

Doris Day: "The really frightening thing about middle age is that you know you'll grow out of it."

Lillian Carter, in her eighties: "Sure I'm for helping the elderly. I'm going to be old myself some day."

Willa Cather: "The dead might as well try to speak to the living as the old to the young."

Henri Estienne: "If youth knew; if age could."

Malcolm Forbes: "After 40, one's face begins to tell more than one's tongue."

Not so fast Malcolm. As Charles Eugster and so many other active-alive-spry seniors are showing us—life, rather than beginning at 40, may in fact kick into gear at 90. But who can wait that long? Best to start working out slowly and steadily with a balanced program now, so you'll robustly hit the nifty 90-plus ground, running and rousting.

Fast forward. Our hero is now 93 years old. He's not resting on his laurels, far from it—he's going for the baubles that would come from winning the "Triple Crown." What he'd have to do is come out on top in rowing, fitness, and athletics. It's enough to turn the average person's hair gray but not Charles's. He insists he has reversed aging with gray hairs on his bod turning brown.

Get outta town! But first come on over and show us more. Encore.

Chapter 41
Does smoking marijuana (pot, grass, weed) make you skinny?

Does smoking, or other substance use, help or hurt weight control?

Does smoking pot make you skinny? A study published in the *American Journal of Epidemiology* (2011) found that if you are a stoner who gets high three times per week, chances are, you will weigh less than peers who don't go for the grass buzz. Who knew rolling a fatty could make you a skinny?

That study surveyed two other studies. In all, about 52,000 Americans came under the pot microscope. In the first study, 22% of non-marijuana smokers were obese compared to 14% who toked; in the second study: 25% versus 17%.

What about the munchies (thanks to cannabinoids)? Surely, after cooking a doobie, one has to have 10 scoops of the hunky-butty, fudgy-nutty, sludgy-banana, creamy-double-flunky, churn-yearn-urn ice cream *to top off* the barbecue chip/ chocolate-chip salad, right?

Maybe the munchies are mitigated by the fact that marijuana is a crop raised without conspicuous labor-saving devices. It is a serious cash crop, but because it is largely illegal, no John Deere harvesters bring in the bounty at season's end. Someone must drag those heavy, bud-laden 8–to 12–foot plants to market.

Hauling that hemp, that Orange Krush over the Hindu Kush, or that home-grown hydroponic dope from the Emerald Triangle in Northern California down to San Francisco, mile after mile, burning all those calories per mile, coupled with losing extra lard through sheer terror —dodging cruisers, choppers, and bandits— is a surefire way to get that weight down, or keep it down. Who could get obese on these beats?

To say that the language this French study uses is wooden is to say that the Amazon rain forest is wet. No matter. The language, dry and near indecipherable though it may be, indicates that more study is needed on this—*light up and lighten up*—relationship between pot and pot bellies.

The study apparently adjusted for sex and age. What, at the same time? Are we talking age of the participants or age of the puffables? The fact is, people of all ages smoke pot. Other than a youngster who has not taken their first drag, or an oldster who has been dragged to the crematorium—once a marijuana smoker, always a marijuana smoker. Just joshing.

As far as sex is concerned, here, the medics are not talking about the well-publicized fear that sex and reefer will allegedly make everyone blind. Rather, they need to adjust their expectations of normal BMI based on whether the study subject is a man or a woman.

Back to the study. Yann le Strat, psychiatrist at the Louis-Mourier Hospital in Colombes, France, led the researchers. No need to read the rest of the mumbo-jumbo to see that these findings can only help those who want to see weed legalized in more states throughout America.

The government, when not sticking its head up its butt, is terribly fat-headed. No doubt the politicians and bureaucrats will continue thundering their jeremiads about marijuana being a "gateway" to cocaine and ecstasy when, duh, everyone knows that money and mental retardation are the actual doorways to that duo.

Moving right along…

Fussbudgets say one must be careful not to draw a cause-and-effect correlation between marijuana use and thinner bodies; in other words, just because there is a direct correlation in a study adjusted for sex and age doesn't mean that someone should draw it.

They obfuscate, mumbling that religious folks smoke less dope (conveniently or confusingly forgetting that marijuana is a sacrament for Church of the Universe). And more significantly in terms of numbers, that religious people are more obese. That's according to a study, Coronary Artery Risk Development in Young Adults, led by Matthew Feinstein (2011). Perhaps it is because praying is a sedentary activity. You have to wonder: wouldn't God-fearing types pray for an acceptable BMI—Body Mass Index? Just asking.

Let's kick the tires on generalization. Let's hit below the belt and declare that some marijuana smokers are not just bong-brained couch potatoes, but are active members of their communities, so long as those communities consist of fellow Frisbee players. Or sprinters. Believe it or not, before testing for performance-enhancing and recreational drugs went crazy, some sprinters would puff a little herb before a training session to deaden the pain from the exertions to come. You don't see a lot of chubby Frisbee players or sprinters do you?

We can be specific here, for the younger set: Don't look to the folks for help on this one. If you ask mom and dad whether you should cook more than the two joints you average daily, chances are they'll drop dead of a heart attack. They don't think you partake at all, according to a 2011 poll from the Mott Children's Hospital. Most parents polled thought that their children used drugs less often than other people's kids, a clear impossibility. It suggests there is a huge incongruence between what the parents think their dears are up to, and what the curs are actually doing.

Should we look to the law and its protectors and enforcers, on all things marijuana? Can we safely assume Alaskan State Troopers, by and large, don't smoke marijuana? Are we agreed? What are we to make of their discovery that—wait for it—marijuana has an odor? (*Weed Times,* August 30, 2011) No. Say it ain't so.

Truth be told, they used the University of Alaska Anchorage Justice Center to snoop around and sniff out their three years worth of haulage to determine that, yes indeed, the weed reeked.

One should not take up marijuana to lose weight, one should take it up for its, ahem, spin-off benefits—but you did not read that here. Though it may have ancillary features that stem obesity, the best way to deal with the latter is, apparently, to drop God like a stone—though you did not read that here either. Marijuana is for recreation, not for reduction. It's for wrecking your life via inhalation; it's not for weight control, though that's a bodacious bonus.

Whatever the tie between weight control and marijuana, one should do with both what one deems best. But perhaps we should all pay heed and adhere to this great maxim, uttered by somebody or other: "The objective in life should not be to arrive at the finish in a pristine condition but to slide sideways across the finish line, belching smoke, leaking oil and worn out."

Put that in your pipe and smoke it.

Chapter 42

Stand on grass: marijuana legalization
or marijuana decriminalization?

Besides starting with the letter C, what do Chicago and Colombia have in common? Both are touting either marijuana decriminalization or marijuana legalization strategies. Are these stoner, boner, bong-headed ideas?

Get a puff of this: Colombia's President, Juan Manuel Santos, called for marijuana legalization globally, with other countries—not his own—leading the way. That may be just as well. Colombia, tragically, is already leading the way in civil wars—it has suffered the longest internecine civil war in a nation's history. No doubt if Colombians pushed this proposal too aggressively in the homeland, internal security would be as incongruous as a politician with a sense of ethics.

Or as Mr. Santos so succinctly put it: "… I would be crucified if I took the first step."

El Presidente may be on to something. Most assuredly, the global and national war on drugs has benefited no one, save for the budget directors of the anti-drug agencies funded to-the-nines for the cause. People, real people, are seemingly hard-wired to screw up their lives and will pop pills, smoke spliffs, or inject idiocies every chance they get, to prove it.

In the USA, marijuana decriminalization in selective jurisdictions might seem a logical first step, as half that nation is on the dole and the other—working—half may be toking up to cope. But starting with Nancy Reagan's "Just Say No" campaign, the States hasn't really had much to offer in the way of practical, doable solutions. (Possibly President Obama could start drone-dropping dynamite on dealers, the way he offs people he's not fond of in far off lands. It isn't community organizing in Chicago, but at least it's a living.)

Aah, Chicago. What's up there?

Recently, Windy City councilmen proposed a local law that would decriminalize possession of small amounts of marijuana, to cut costs and save police time for more serious crimes.

There might be one problem with *any* legalization/decriminalization gambit: If governments worldwide—not known for measureable efficiencies at the local, state, national, or supranational level—were to get their clammy-grabby, grubby, ham-fisted hands on marijuana—they would probably, through typical malfeasance and tiresome negligence, *dry up the bud supply*. No easy task with a weed, I grant you, but look how governments in America control education—and look how hard it is to get a good education anywhere.

But even with government initiatives, there's always an exception that proves the rule. If, as a government, you want to grow marijuana for medicinal purposes, you could do a lot worse than growing the stuff in an old copper mine.

Talk about an underground industry. Way back in 2000 or so, the federal government of Canada, under the auspices and somewhat good offices of a minion of the Dominion, created the "Rock Garden" to grow marijuana for medical purposes. We are told, "Health Minister Allan Rock went down for a look Thursday and said the 43-day-old plants were almost as tall as he is —six feet…" (*Cannabis News*, August 2, 2011)

But that ain't the main deal. The main deal is that marijuana has over 400 active chemical compounds, more than the USA has I.O.U's. Some of these compounds may in fact aid in the treatment of muscle pain, insomnia, and digestive system disorders. Definitely, good reefer will get you higher than a Michael Jordan slam dunk, but generally speaking, cannabis differs from some substances in that it doesn't breed and abet wanton violence—unless you are a purveyor, procurer, promoter, pusher, or peddler of it.

Maybe taking out the middleman—the disruptive, slimy, grimy seller—and replacing him with a rude and rigid fat-cat unionized government bureaucrat, is the way to go. Sure the service will suck, the reefer retail store will forever be on strike, and its employees will protest and picket your garden patch should you scab and try to compete with their demon weed. But hey—at least they won't shoot you if they don't like the look of your money or your face. They'll tax you to death—but that's legal.

And here's a big plus, not for the consumer but for the government employees entrusted with legal reefer. The end-user will be gouged and screwed over because the administrator, seeder, grower, distributor, and caterer—being part of the 114% of all governmental jobs that are magically mandated union ones—will take home gobs in huge salaries and bonanza benefits—and that money has to come from you, the schlep smoker toker.

Whether getting knifed in the back economically feels socially, morally, and ethically preferable to hearing about poor ganja growers in Colombia getting exploited, drastically and dramatically, up the yin-yang is a tough call.

But the governments of the day haven't had to make tough policy calls. Particularly in the US of A, they have taken refuge in seeing marijuana as a cultural failing, something to be shunned.

Crazy, that. Dopers may have hygiene problems but are they as big a problem as drunk drivers who leave messy, bloody, unclean-hygiene highway scenes? And that tragic play, so long as booze is legal, is sadly here to stay.

But hope may be on the way for marijuana activists. Witness 4/20, the global day on which potheads everywhere gather to protest crazy marijuana laws. Canada's best west, left city Vancouver, now sees about 20,000 turn out to protest and puff. Amazingly, the police arrest none of the protesters. The police are suffering from a collective case of glaucoma, one would guess. Hold it! Doesn't marijuana help treat glaucoma?

Apologies, got off track there… but the track, inevitably if not inexorably, seems to lead to a loosening of reefer regulations, if regular folks' pot perceptions are any indication. In Colorado and in the state of Washington, ballots to legalize marijuana passed. In the USA and Canada, polled together, Angus Reid pollsters found (December 29, 2011) that two-thirds of those surveyed agreed with the statement that the "War on Drugs" was a failure.

Nevertheless, decriminalized or legalized marijuana in the social mainstream, as opposed to specific exceptions such as "medical marijuana", seems a tough row to hoe: politicians pander everywhere to "values." These values are shouted from every rooftop and street corner, and they don't go hand in hand with grass. One issue for politicians is that the people who turn out to vote, generally, are not lazy, hazy, dozy toker smokers—so it would seem that legal marijuana is not, except for the avant-garde jurisdictions mentioned above, in the electoral cards, no matter what Chicago thinks. Colombia, historically, has been a haven of criminality but it doesn't compare to Chicago's cesspool of vice. Realistically, why would anyone look to either that city, or that country, as beacons to follow and as bastions of advice to heed—for weed? This issue will be with us for a while, it seems.

Chapter 43
Systemic abuse of painkiller drugs epidemic in USA

"Epidemic" in the United States? That's what the BBC News headline (November 1, 2011) basically blares. Should it come as a surprise? If there was no prescription painkiller abuse—now *that* would be news.

Nevertheless, it might be wise to probe just why Americans are going off the deep end left, right, and center, to ease pain, real or imagined, from their lives. First, it's not like the USA isn't going through painful times right now. For one thing, Americans had to suffer through the interminable Republican presidential contender debates that showed no signs of slowing down or improving in intellectual quality. That had to hurt. (Not as much as it hurt Mitt Romney to now be a footnote in the history of presidential wannabes.)

Of course, these gab sessions are merely a sidebar to the non-stop class war conducted by the hectoring teleprompter President, the fellow that ruined private industry job creation, Barack Obama. With him and the GOP in campaign mode until the 6 November 2012 presidential election, could we blame the commoners for tuning them out by any means possible? (Even after his win, President Obama is still on the campaign circuit. Where *is* the off switch? Where *are* those painkillers?)

Seriously, with the wars, battles, "kinetic military actions," conflagrations, scuffles—call them what you will, in Afghanistan, Iraq, and late of Libya—just how many soldiers live under the thumbscrews of legally prescribed narcotics?

And what of the Occupy Wall Street (OWS) crowd? With the weather turning faster than a Tasmanian devil on steroids, surely that motley crew needed help to cope with the most recent drastic climate change—the onset of winter. And such hassles might force the loutish loiterers in Oakland, dealing with the long arm of the law, to bum and cadge for over-the-top and under-the-counter prescriptions.

And factor in an aging population into the mix. Many seniors use several prescription drugs, quite legitimately, to treat chronic illnesses. That, however, can prove a "gateway" to abuse of legal drugs, which are often cheap or free, depending on one's income or health plan.

Americans may be silly, frightening, alarmingly friendly, or disarmingly unfathomable—but they're not dumb. The BBC One story says that Americans take painkillers more than they abuse heroin or cocaine combined. This is intended, one would surmise, to shock the reader—but it should do exactly the opposite.

Have you bought cocaine or heroin lately? Of course you haven't. Do you know, theoretically, what you would fork out per gram to "speedball" these solutions? Probably about a hundred dollars per gram for the tootskie and more for the smack. America's economy is in a free fall. It hasn't hit rock bottom like Greece but with nearly half the populace on government assistance, few will be laying out their entitlement dollars for any rock soon. Where will they turn for a palliative for their personal psychological problems, aromatherapy?

Forget counseling. Think. That's really expensive and who needs a shrink to confirm what you already suspect—that you are a complete loser, a naff, a twink, a dolt? So a jolt of legal painkillers is the order of the day.

But before you succumb to the temptations of a legally available elixir to brighten your life (or at least to dim its blight)—think twice. Yes, painkillers do work as advertised—but they may also work as unadvertised too. Fool around with prescription amounts at your peril, for you'll find not only that the overwhelming pain has gone, but that the bunion, the scrape, and the cut are no longer bugging you. You have woken up one day to discover that *you are dead*.

Consider: A report published by the Centers for Disease Control and Prevention (CDC) says fatalities caused by narcotic pain relievers have more than tripled in the last 10 years—reaching about 40 deaths a day.

Drugs, booze—whatever—have been bandied about since the times of Pharaohs. They aren't going away soon. *Dancing with the Stars* is a great escapist placebo—but it can't run forever (although 13 years in the USA is a good stint)—so alternatives to painkiller abuse might be needed.

Physician heal thyself. Huh? If you are concerned that doping up is taking you, or a friend or family member down, it would be best to look to personal solutions as a means to stymie the drug drip. Don't look to the government. Drug law in the USA is a patchwork in progress, legislated largely by individual states. Each state is as different from the other as is Pluto from Jupiter. Think of 52 states (parents) telling you how to live your life in varying tones of effectiveness and intent. By the time those jurisdictions, especially senior citizen-friendly Florida, get a handle on pill mills, you might be a goner.

A quick peek at the top 10 American consumer complaints in 2011, according to ABC 15.com, explains why painkillers are so popular (quite apart from their easing physical pain). The beefs with cars, utilities, debt, home improvements/construction, retail sales, services, Internet sales, for example, are not incidental; they are the DNA of every sentient person's life. If the basics suck, if everything around you stinks—why wouldn't you want to, metaphorically at least, go numb and dumb with painkillers?

Fifty-five hundred folks start misusing prescription painkillers every day. So says Pamela Hyde, administrator for the Substance Abuse and Mental Health Services Administration. By year's end, that comes to 2,007,500 of us who will add to the gazillions who are, intentionally or unintentionally, already ruining their lives.

Can Americans stop abusing painkillers? Possibly. Probably. People can, and do, change. It won't be easy. Any drug, prescription or recreational, is hard to quit—it quite often means not only stopping the drug but dumping friends associated with the drug. And let's not even talk about how to handle the souse, shooter-upper, or pill-swilling spouse. Nevertheless what are the alternatives? Ironically, painkiller overindulgence makes life painful, what with self-esteem lower than a basset hound's nose to the ground. Why not wake up and smell the painkiller drug abuse epidemic, American citizenry?

Chapter 44

Can steroids really help you win, and
lose (weight) at the same time?

Giving nature a nudge—Is it worth the risks?

What beats character, conduct, civility, and conscience when cash and celebrity are up for grabs? In sports, it's the illegal, surreptitious use of steroids.

It's ironic. Steroids have not been uncommon in the gladiator sports of pro wrestling and football. It takes balls to risk life and limb on anabolic steroids. You might get your perfunctory 15 minutes of fame, but then again you might get everlasting notoriety for testicles shriveled to the size of chickpeas. Please. But men, take heart. If you do dabble and dipstick with steroids, your new, larger breasts will compensate for your old, smaller balls.

In "History of Doping in Sport" (*Journal of Sports Studies*, 2001), Charles E. Yesalis and Michael S. Bahrke mention the Zanes, the bronze statues of Zeus, king of the gods, which lined the athletes' way into the ancient Olympics. These statues, funded from fines for bribery, lying, and cheating, sat atop low pedestals and were thought to take note of athletes who broke Olympic rules back in 776 BC–394 AD.

Want to be an Adonis? Go honest. Don't take steroids, eat sensibly, and work out strenuously. See where these strategies get you. And by not taking steroids you'll accrue these advantages too:

1) You will not have to testify before a supercilious, suspicious US congressional committee on why you were able to hit 90 homers, up slightly from the 8 round trippers whacked the year before.

2) You will avoid being disingenuous, dissembling like Popeye-forearmed Mark McGwire, who didn't want to talk about the past, yet somehow hoped

to be a positive influence for the future! Thereby you will avoid being the most derided person in the room—in and of itself a near impossible task, given that the room is stocked with self-important, playing-to-the-press, pasty, whey-faced, puerile politicians.

3) You'll avoid buying steroids on the street from the sales ringer-upper, a pimply 14-year-old whose calf muscles are twice the size of your thighs. You'll avoid gutlessness when the wheeler dealer intimidates you to pay twice the price.

4) You'll avoid the guilty chills and sweaty thrills that come from toting huge brown paper bags filled with Dianabol ("Dbol")—not even realizing that, not only have your teammates not figured it out, everyone thinks you're toting weird pornographic S&M ball and chain accessories around.

5) You'll avoid having to give back gold medals that were mendaciously, shamefully won. Marion Jones, come on down! And bring those three gold and two bronze medals from the 2000 Sydney Olympics with you!

6) You'll avoid so-called friends leaking your possible steroid use to the media. You'll also avoid steroid abuse-induced pain every time you take a leak.

True, taking "pumpers," "stackers," and "gym candy" has earned some wrestlers and football players palatial homes, trophy spouses, and entourages. But it has also earned them urns: And all they had to do for it was sacrifice their lives to steroids while alive, so they could enjoy eternity being dead, while dead.

It's also earned some heavy steroid takers a wide berth in public, not because of their deeply veined formidable muscles, but because of their deeply seated, over-heated, contemptible foaming and frothing. All us innocents would love to see you forego the fomenting, put the pit bull muzzle back on, and please, pretty please, please slither back into your cage. We are trying to catch up on the latest news—and, little do we know, the next segment might involve high school kids you're selling to.

Heard it on the grapevine that teens are abusing steroids too. Seriously, in 2006 the Grapevine–Colleyville school district in Texas started random testing for drugs (including steroids) for those "students who participate in sports and other extra-curricular activities, from drama and debate to cheerleading and choir."

Steroids for choir? Sing it ain't so.

In New Jersey, those tempted to take steroids are singing the blues, for that state now has obligatory tests for performance-enhancing drugs for high schoolers in all sports.

Kids, try not to succumb to peer pressure and don't become an AAS user. AAS user? It means don't take *androgenic anabolic steroids*.

One of the major reasons why the vast majority of school districts do not do random or mandatory testing, apart from constitutional issues around privacy rights and unreasonable searches, is the prohibitive cost. A cocaine-tootski test may be in the neighborhood of $20. For steroids, triple or quadruple that. With budgets stretched tighter than a diaper on an incontinent elephant, schools find that it makes more sense, to save cents, to screen kids for weed and blow via urine, hair, or saliva samples than it does to screen for steroids.

Illegal steroids, as opposed to steroids such as testosterone that your body produces naturally, are not only dangerous to the chooser-user-loser, but are, as star pitcher Roger Clemens' saga demonstrates, a blight on the user's aura. Imagine the ignominy of having such a disreputable, disgusting institution like Congress (again), with a reputation miles below a snake and a hair's width above a cockroach, accusing you of taking steroids. (Roger, incidentally, was acquitted. It only took five short years.) But he wasn't alone. Congress has held nine hearings on the spectacle-debacle of steroids in sports as of early 2013.

Do you remember how Sylvester Stallone got busted a few short years ago? "Rocky Balboa" was down for the count and counted out in Australia, the Land Down Under.(AP) Sydney reported,

Sylvester Stallone was convicted yesterday (May 21, 2007) of importing restricted muscle-building hormones, which he told customs officials he needed to stave off the feelings of aging and give his 60-year-old body a boost.

They found a total of 48 vials of the steroid [HGH (Human Growth Hormone)] after they raided Stallone's hotel room, limousine and private jet.

In a letter to the court in which he apologized for a "terrible mistake", Stallone said he had taken the drugs for years to treat a medical condition that he didn't disclose.

What medical condition? A peculiar predilection for making the same picture over and over again, with different titles?

Again, AP tells us that "Citing testimony from Stallone's Beverly Hills-based doctor, [New South Wales state deputy Chief Magistrate] Paul Cloran "found that Stallone had been using the testosterone legally under medical supervision, although he had failed to declare it to customs officials."

Sylvester Stallone needs extra testosterone? Moving right along, back in time…

It's hard to say which was worse in the late 1970s, the advent of steroid use in sports or the popularity of disco dancing anywhere. On reflection, disco was worse. At least steroid users had tangible goals. Folks, young and old, then and now, snort, swallow, or shoot steroids to build lean muscles, delay fatigue, engender euphoria, allow for faster-than-normal recovery times from injury, beat the tar out of non-steroid competitors, and scare the bejeebers out of their chemist drug-masking magicians. All in the hope of conjuring, in pursuit of Olympian heights (*Citius, Altius, Fortius* , that is,"Faster, Higher, Stronger"), the undetectable drug cocktail combinations that sully the sports of today and will stain the sports of tomorrow.

While we're on the topic of soiled and spoiled, did you know that a popular method of taking steroids by the week or month, or up to three months with breaks in between, is known as cycling? A derivative of this method is known as the Tour de France.

Just kidding. Maybe.

For good measure, to compound the solution (and the problem), many athletes mix steroids with stimulants and depressants. This seems counterintuitive because uppers and downers taken at the same time would cancel each other out, no?

Stuff it, you say? You think, "Me taking steroids hurts nobody but myself." Physically, you're probably right, except for when you stupidly whack mom and dad silly when they refuse to front you your college money for next year's steroid supply. But mentally you bum out all those amateur rivals who play clean. (Let's leave the clean pros out of this; any sad feelings they harbor are ameliorated by astronomical paydays.)

Steroids, and the deceptions that arise from their illegal use, bring to mind the Russian proverb: With lies you may go ahead in the world—but you can never go back. (But apparently, sometimes you *can* get back your balls. They'll grow back to a more normal size if you stop taking steroids.)

Maybe.

Chapter 45
Lawsuit filed after woman dies following lap-band surgery

Four obese people chose this type of surgery as a shortcut to losing weight, and they are dead. Is the Lap-Band procedure at fault? One widely reported case involved Laura Faitro who died following the Lap-Band procedure. Her bereaved husband sued, among others, the Valley Surgical Center, which is affiliated with 1-800-GET-THIN . There are no winners here, save for the lawyers, eventually—but nobody likes lawyers, so count them as losers too. But if everybody else plays their cards wrong, all should be barren, bitter, broke, and buried at the end.

Before we sift through the remains of the Laura Faitro case, perhaps we should look at what this Lap-Band procedure is. Here are the guts of the operation:

Lap-Band or gastric banding is done using laparoscopic surgery. A surgeon, after inserting a camera into the stomach, uses the visual feedback to position a band made of inflatable silicone in the abdomen. The surgeon makes small incisions, using instruments with long handles, to create a small, circular tunnel behind the stomach. He then inserts the gastric band through the tunnel, and locks the band around the stomach.

The band forms a pouch at the top of the stomach. The pouch acts as a new, front-line stomach. It can hold about one-half a cup of food where the average stomach holds six cups. It fills quickly and sends a message to the brain that says: "Hey I'm stuffed down here. No more food." The food that was already eaten then passes slowly into the lower part of the stomach.

The Lap-Band system got FDA approval back in 2001. It's complicated, as most surgery is, but it has one advantage (at least when folks aren't dying ostensibly because of it) in that it does not necessitate any cutting or removal of the digestive system. You can also do an "Edit-Undo." It is reversible. Hopefully the weight doesn't come whooshing back, but that's another story.

So far so good. Reports are glowing—many patients lose weight, feel confident, and get their lives back, for better or for worse.

But worse can happen if the Faitro lawsuit is any indication. Gastric bandings can have, ahem, drastic landings. Laura Faitro was the fourth to die in California following the Lap-Band Procedure.

But setting aside the sad situation of fatalities for the moment, who is eligible for the Lap-Band? Well, being near morbidly obese is not all. You must have flunked, for six months, medically supervised dietary therapy. Besides being 100 pounds or so above your ideal weight, you must show awareness that the post-surgical period will be painful and that the future will involve big changes to diet and portion sizes, if long-term triumph is to result.

In Laura Faitro's case, however, it seems as though everyone is blameless and blameworthy simultaneously; it just depends on who is speaking about whom. Egregiously, the lawyer representing the Valley Surgical Center, Robert Silverman, essentially blamed Laura Faitro's life for her death: "It would appear that Ms. Faitro died of non-Lap Band related issues due to her extremely poor overall health condition," he said. Of course he could very well be bang on. The Lap-Band was intended for patients who exhibit certain co-morbidities, that is, diseases that accompany serious obesity. But one inconvenient truth for lawyer Silverman and his client is the ghastly fact that Faitro's liver was lacerated three times during the Lap-Band procedure. The husband, properly pissed at having his wife die just five days after the operation, has sued not only the aforesaid Valley Surgical Center but also the 1-800-GET-THIN, Simi Valley Hospital, and doctors at both institutions.

The surgeon who performed the operation, Dr. Ihsan Shamaan, states in a sworn deposition that he was pressured to commit perjury by Michael and Julian Omidi, the California-based brothers behind the 1-800-GET-THIN signs. The surgeon also admits to lacerating Faitro's liver during the procedure.

Clearly, not all these organizations and individuals can be equally responsible for Laura Faitro's death but due to the mounds of pre-trial publicity, everyone will be tarred. The fumbling for position is reminiscent of a crowd of male red-sided garter snakes wrapping themselves around a female snake, hoping to mate.

But at least the snakes are not slimy.

The lawsuit was settled in early 2013, with the terms kept confidential. However, we do know that Mrs. Faitro's death certificate listed heart failure as the cause of death, with liver laceration and morbid obesity as contributing factors. The take-home point is that if you get to the point where you are 100 pounds overweight, not only is your condition life-threatening, but so is the surgery, potentially.

Chapter 46
Robotic surgery and remote surgery

Eventually, whether healthy or sickly, some of us will need an operation of one type or another. Could it be done by a robot?

Let's say you are in Strasbourg, France. You are tooling around in the city center—which has been designated a World Heritage Site by the UN—when, all of a sudden, you have a serious gall bladder attack, and you need your gallbladder removed.

But your favorite doctor, who does the cholecystectomy operation to remove gall bladders like it's going out of style, is tied up in New York.

No problem. Strike up the band. Remote robotic surgery is at hand. Dr. Jacques Marescaux and Dr. Michel Gagner can perform on you from America—in this "Lindbergh operation"—while you hang (metaphorically) in France. Later, when the operation goes off without a hitch and friends marvel at your gallbladderlessness and ask who did the deed, you proclaim:

ZEUS!

Robotic surgery, or telesurgery has been kicking around in various shapes and forms since the late 1990s and the jury is in—with mixed reviews, leaning to positive. Patients and surgeons love it, but the bean counters of the medical world are much less infatuated.

Patients love it because their recovery is faster. There's also a lot less pain, and less of the scary scarring that is typical with traditional hard-core cutting and separating techniques.

The Greek god Zeus had his fingers in a lot of pies and the medical robot Zeus, not to be outdone, has three arms. It was developed by Computer Motion, an American company now called Intuitive Surgical.

You may think this stuff is far-out, space-cadet material, and you wouldn't be wrong. NASA had been tinkering with robotic arms and worked with Computer Motion to develop the AESOP arm. Computer Motion married advanced technology with a gift for catchy names. It boasts a control center called HERMES and a telecollaboration system called SOCRATES.

Robot surgeons are the baseball relievers for the medical field. Like a starting pitcher whose arm is about to fall off, a surgeon gets plenty tired doing traditional surgery. Having a robot perform these tasks while a surgeon pulls the strings behind a Wizard-of-Oz curtain is a big relief.

Of course the difference is that the starting-pitcher surgeon has to figure out how to work the goldarn thing, but school's right up their powerhouse alley so…

How, in a nutshell, does remote robotic surgery work? Through telepresence. Telepresence is epitomized by videoconferencing.

The range of possibilities for remote surgery is vast. Say you're a soldier, barging around in a foreign land, and you get barged into. And the medical know-how there isn't quite up to snuff. This is a perfect opportunity for remote surgery to work medical magic.

Here, there, or anywhere, before you can say *presto!*, robotic surgery is starting to be used as a key component of heart surgery, kidney transplants, liver resection, catheter guidance, and hernia repair—and a whole host of gynecological procedures besides.

Women need not fear gangly artificial odds and ends poking around down there; most real-live men are pretty mechanical as they perfunctorily go through the motions when it comes to all deeds in this below-the-equator zone anyway, so the adjustment will be negligible.

Let's elevate the conversation…

Have you heard of da Vinci surgery? It is a big player in the field. Traditional knowledge and practices have come a long way from the cruel days of yore, using ice to wash away pain. Now booze is used to slosh away pain. Similarly, surgery has graduated from simple, brutal, ritual amputation to, well, basically three options. They are: traditional surgery that makes huge cuts, laparoscopic surgery, and keyhole surgery, which is a whole lot better because of its small incisions. But unfortunately, it is limited to the abdomen as its main theater of operations. But now there is a fourth option: Non-invasive robotic surgery. The da Vinci surgical system, if their Web site is anything to go by, is a leader.

While small cuts are the cat's meow, the cost of robotic operators will scratch a hole in hospital budgets. A robotic surgical unit costs anywhere from a million to two million, plus. (On the bright side, the machines don't put in for overtime or claim dog-ate-the-homework sick days.) The quest for innovation is a wonderful one, and while the advantages seem obvious, negatives may crop up after more studies arm wrestle the merits of robots.

For sure, the known, quite exorbitant expenses, give us pause to puke. It cost, for instance, more than €1 million to do the "Lindbergh" gallbladder removal on a woman in France in 2002, the most expensive surgery in history at the time.

Let's pretend we are governments who blithely and blindly run up deficits faster than the Bellagio and the MGM Grand run up winnings. Cost, therefore, is not an issue. Picture instead a doctor with his head in what looks to be suction bowl, peering into a new-fangled arcade contraption. His arms and fingers are flying, fidgeting, and finagling like your favorite concert pianist. His feet are feverishly tapping, toeing, and tooling around to his own beat or, better yet, the patient's. And—in the next room or in a land across the ocean, octopus arms ending with little tweezers—all triple jointed—are each doing their thing.

It's like Robert Downey Jr. and his *Iron Man* suit going to town on you separately.

And don't worry if the doctor "drank lunch": tremors are a thing of the past with robotic surgery, and a blurry—or sharp—eye is *magnified by 10* using this technology.

It's great to be on the cutting edge of medical history and heroics, huh? Perhaps obesity surgery, if needed, will one day be safer.

Now let's hope we never need any of this stuff!

Chapter 47
Sitting most of the day means health problems

Work and School Fitness—Risks and Rewards

You!—you there, sitting down on the job at work! Stand up for your own good. Tons of evidence says sitting down on the job literally stops you from burning calories, for one thing, and creates certain cancers, diabetes, and heart disorders, for another. If you can live with those debilities, sit back, relax, and smell the roses while you can.

And while we all know that television can be educational (or at least keep the adults entertained and the kids busy), know this also: Watching TV, sitting for hours on end, will grant you not only a smattering of knowledge but a short shelf life, aka early death. Too bad, so sad. You want proof?

Seventeen thousand Canadians (strictly, 17,013) were human guinea pigs in a 12-year study on the effects of prolonged sitting on Canadians from eighteen to ninety years of age. There was significantly greater mortality from all causes among study participants who spent a great deal of time sitting, *irrespective of whether they were physically active during their leisure time.* In other words, sitting down all day at work is bad for you even if you compensate by getting some exercise in after work. The bottom line, so to speak, is that you just should not be sitting down so much. (American College of Sports Medicine, 2006; Katzmarzyk, P. T. et al. 2009. "Sitting time and mortality from all causes, cardiovascular disease, and cancer." *Medicine and Science in Sports and Exercise* 41: 998–1005).

We don't have to sit down all the time just to get work done. After sitting down and working through these last three paragraphs for ten minutes, I have stopped the sedentary scribbling, stood up, and started shuffling about. And good on me for keeping on the move, for every half hour or so on the go is crucial to stretching out that otherwise short, seated shelf life.

Fifty-five per cent. Using data collected from 2003 to 2004, that is the estimated time of their *waking* day, that Americans—adults and kids—spend on their keester, whether eating, working, or watching TV. It is, however, sitting on the job that causes health problems for workers—and sometimes, passengers, perhaps because the workplace limits movement more. Passengers? Say what?

Yes passengers. Apparently, in 2011, an air traffic controller at Reagan International Airport fell asleep on the job, and two passenger planes had to parlay a landing on their own. If the controller had made it a point to get up and move about every 15 minutes or so, he might not be so likely to snooze, with the risk that others might perish…

Here are more horrid facts against sitting down during the whole working day. The vaunted phrase, "studies have shown," earns its keep here: Three life-limiting conditions that can result from prolonged sitting are stiff necks, varicose veins, and numbness in the legs. They won't kill you, but they take the fun out of living.

Obesity triggered by prolonged sitting may lead to inherited problems as well. For obese women, for example, it may help to get off that seat, if only to keep the procreation of the species going. It seems obese women have daughters who are less fertile than their non-obese counterparts, according to a 2011 study in the journal *Endocrinology* (Jaspreet Virk, *The Money Times,* March 24, 2011).

Let's not take this sitting down. If we stay seated, knowing now the fatal facts that will befall us, we may at least want to keep track of the length of the periods in which we and our kids sit, if only to set aside, or better yet defer or delay, a periodic death sentence.

This isn't rocket science. One article breathlessly asks: What can be done to prevent prolonged sitting? Er, um, huh… get *up*? Would that be an answer?

At least rock. You are better to rock in a rocking chair at work, for your legs are doing some pushing, however piffling and pedestrian the amounts. Will the boss go for this? Do you have stairs at the office, or at home? You could use them as an inexpensive exertion—they don't break, and as far as your personal residence goes, don't cost a penny, other than the rent or mortgage paid on them.

So get back on the beam, get back on track, and beat that sitting-down, slumping-around, slow-death sneak attack.

Chapter 48
Work walk

Hey sitters, have I got fantastic news for you. Your weight problems are *so* over. Why? Well, because I have seen the future and it is us, you and me, marching away while at work—for eight, count 'em eight, hours per day on the FitWork Walkstation.

In 2008, intrepid *Globe & Mail* reporter Rebecca Dube checked out the apparatus for our benefit ("Burning & Earning"). She walked 16 kilometers on the treadmill-cum-desk, as she calls it. While her legs were mush afterwards, if she had been obese and worked with this station daily, she would have lost 44 to 66 pounds by year's end. You'd almost want to gain the weight first, to see if this really holds true, wouldn't you?

No? All right.

Here is the long and short of it. The machine retails (2008 dollars, don't forget) for around $4,500. The gizmo is made in Michigan, and there is a philosophy behind it.

Neat huh? A philosophy. No, NEAT *is* the philosophy. The acronym stands for non-exercise activity thermogenesis. Thermogenesis means giving off heat, in other words, burning calories. NEAT encompasses all of our daily activities that would usually be sedentary, that is, activities apart from gym sessions, walking the dogs, buying the newspaper, chasing the kids, and so on. James Levine, a Mayo Clinic researcher, found in a 2005 study that "NEAT influences our weight more than the time we spend formally exercising."

Now if you had one of these at your workplace, say in a department of 20 people, and each of you used the Walkstation for 20 minutes per day (a much more reasonable starting point than Rebecca's 16 kilometers), *presto!*, the department would shrink.

But shrink in a just way, through sizing down. That beats downsizing and "right-sizing," when office co-workers get the chop. Our goal here is reduced clothing sizes, not staff sizes.

In Canada some food manufacturing, Internet, and financial services firms ordered the machine, and the testimonials from American firms on the company's Web site are glowing.

One drawback is that serious brain-boggling work like analyzing, drafting reports, and on-the-fly, by-the-seat-of-your-pants problem-solving skills are hard to practice while you are on this machine, even though your maximum speed is 2 miles per hour and you don't break a sweat. But reading e-mails, filing attachments, general office housekeeping chores, and even yakking on the phone are all doable.

(And with the low sound, high torque motor, and the optional privacy screen working as they should, your fellow employees won't even know you've been sauntering all day, though they might wonder what's up if your weight is way down six months hence.)

Nobody does better research for you than you do. There are lots of work-walking blogs to check out, to ponder the merits of walking while you work. (Please arrange to have a benevolent employer who'll spring for the cash to buy these machines while you're at it.)

Imagine losing weight at work instead of losing your mind. Makes you almost want to get out of bed in the morning on a Monday...

Okay, a Friday.

Chapter 49
Work walk—will liability issues crush the idea?

Good heavens. Just as we were thinking of investing in work-walking futures, or at least pondering taking up this exercise in the here and now, some observers are squawking that with work-walking comes lousy work results and resultant injuries. These injuries are not caused by irate bosses peeved at declining productivity, but by the use of these machines.

In a recent article in *MarketWatch,* we are told that, at least in 2011 in the USA, detriments such as decreased typing accuracy and speed, and poorer hand-mouse dexterity resulted, with home and office treadmill injuries comprising 37% of exercise equipment accidents (Jen Wieczner, "Is your ergonomic desk trying to kill you?", January 29, 2013).

Proponents may counter that they experience the benefits of "feeling less lethargic," a soft, anecdotal, hard-to-quantify description, if there ever was one. How can that platitude stand up against the hard revelations about Achilles tendon pain (albeit the accounts of the pain are from online community banter)? Now, what if other stats are compiled that show decreased absenteeism, a hard number that definitely impacts the corporate bottom line? Perhaps the impact of the joint injuries that—manufacturers say—are due to initial overuse of these new office gadgets will be dissipated somewhat.

While the thrill of these machines in the workplace dims with time, like office romances, there isn't much doubt that sales have soared for TreadDesk, bringing in, if not a pretty penny in net profit, at least a whole lot more of dimes in gross revenue. According to CEO Jerry Carr, TreadDesk sold 2,800 workstations in 2012—50 times more than when it launched in 2006.

And another thing is a sure bet too: If workplace injuries do rise because of the use of such machines, there will be pain of another sort: lawsuits and increased company insurance premiums. "Companies investing in the walk-at-work movement could expose themselves to employees filing cumulative trauma claims," workers' compensation expert Paul Braun, managing direct with Aon Global Risk Consulting, told *Risk & Insurance Magazine* (December 13, 2011).

Basically, work-walker and employer beware. There probably is some benefit to such machinery in the workplace. But common sense means not walking for hours on end throughout the workday, and listening to your body. And making doubly sure you wash up after a good sweat could also go a long way in maintaining a healthy, harmonious (and odor-free) workspace for all.

Chapter 50
The Olympics and your health

(This piece was written back in June 2007 but still makes the cut today, what with the Canadian government showing no signs of cutting back its Cabinet fat.)

Canada will be blessed with the 2010 Winter Olympics, to be held in Vancouver, British Columbia, and the federal government, led by the Conservative Party of Canada, wants to piggyback on them. It has decided to create a non-official Olympic event centered on obesity.

From what I understand, the roads that lead to official Olympic events, like the slalom and downhill, are questionable in quality. On July 31, 2008, the *Vancouver Sun* detailed how a vital route to Whistler (Highway 99) was felled by a rock slide. It was to be out of commission for an estimated four days. A *National Post* story said large machinery looked like a toy compared to the boulders.

Perhaps the government should concentrate on ensuring ease of access to these and other events. But then again, that doesn't sound like nearly so much fun as poking around in the pantries of its citizenry.

At any rate, Tony Clement is the Health Minister for Canada, and he figures that everybody tuning in to the games will be in a fitness mode. Apparently, he cannot imagine the possibility that they'll be sprawled on the couch with the remote, beer, and popcorn at hand.

"We've got some other things that are gearing up that use the Winter Olympics as a way to get back into people's households on fitness issues," he told media.

What are these other things? They sound ominously, perhaps purposely, vague.

An earlier Canadian Prime Minister, Pierre Elliott Trudeau, once said the government had no business in the bedrooms of the nation and I, for the life of me, can't recall when we asked it to drop into our dens instead.

Nevertheless, Mr. Clement's clarion call to badger Canadians on fitness might lend new meaning to the phrase "fit" governance.

Say what?

The Canadian government's Cabinet, of which Clement is a member, is bloated blob, hovering at 31 members. There are seven other Ministers who are not allowed in the cabinet (maybe they are too big to fit in.) In 2007 Canada had approximately

33 million citizens eligible for federal intrusiveness; the USA, an estimated 301 million. America, with *9 times* the population, fighting wars here, there, and everywhere, makes do with a tight-knit, kick-ass mob of about 18 cabinet ministers.

Maybe the Canadian government should shed some weight off its own behind before getting in front, and in the face, of its folks.

Chapter 51
Witness kids fitness

It's not easy being a kid these days. Especially a fit kid. Why? Various jurisdictions have fitted kids with proverbial straitjackets, banning trampolines here, banishing tobogganing there, and outlawing fun everywhere. Or so it seems. So, as mentioned, kids retreat to such safe havens as the video domain, where they play for days—and get fat.

What's with that?

Most parents mean well, even if they've hardly the time to keep track of time, let alone ensure their youngsters get quality (and quantity) physical fitness in a fun format. Undoubtedly, every mom and dad wants their progeny to start out like George Atkinson, who scaled the Seven Summits (the highest peaks of the seven continents) *at 16*, and to age—well, to age like Charles Eugster, who is still turning heads (and blowing minds) with chin ups, *at 90 plus*.

One thing's for sure. It's not happening. Kids are getting fatter by the moment and now politicians have picked up the apparent slack where parents, theoretically, have dropped the ball. In Chicago some schools banned homemade lunches. In Malaysia kids are graded by their Body Mass Index. Restaurants throughout the USA, increasingly hector, pester, and lecture kids via published calorie counts for meals. Research indicates that kids, being clued in, tune out. Now this is not to say that one should binge on McDonalds' Big Macs, but surely one doesn't go to a fast food restaurant to vegan out either, does one? Scare is everywhere; answers are nowhere.

Do the fitness industry and health clubs have roles to play? In fairness, they have carved out niches. Kids are offered a growing choice of sports activities, and motor skill-building machines to discover, learn, and excel with. But parents and mentors can't sit on their hands willy-nilly, farming out responsibilities to third parties. The kids must be cajoled to shake a leg at home too (in the nicest affirmative, inclusive way) because, as studies have shown, sitting is a flab builder, whether in front of the TV or the computer screen. Zero calories are burned whilst sitting. Also, video games apparently goose up appetites for snacks, definitely a dastardly double whammy.

Of course, parents—and schools, particularly schools, shouldn't go off the deep end and punish kids through—say push-ups. Remember the story of Donell Dixon? He was the 13-year-old who chose push-up purgatory at school and ended up in the hospital (*ABC Action News*, March 25, 2011). So now that approach has hit the fan. A balance between pusillanimity and poking must be found. Let's call the middle ground persuasion. What is to be done? Should one cajole the kid outdoors to imitate Thor, and heave the hammer and train with a kettlebell? Sure, if the kid is old enough, if kettlebell and hammer-heaving techniques have been taught—and if all the neighbors' houses are infilled with foam.

Wealth creation isn't taught easily. Many parents will not have the dough for freestyle skiing, and there may not be any facilities nearby in any event. But are there venues for activities that require little equipment? Soccer and volleyball come to mind. Both are great for speed, skill, strength, and stamina. Believe it or not, weight training for youngsters is growing rapidly in popularity, epitomized by gymnast-weightlifter, little he-man, Giuliano Stroe, who broke two world records for vertical push-ups by the time he was six.

But if the opposite trend to pudgy kids persists, pretty soon fat farms like the California Wellspring Academy will be bursting at the seams everywhere.

Governments have been trying to find a middle way between wanton intrusiveness and willful ignorance. In Canada, for example, Prime Minister Stephen Harper has been trying to trim up the tykes via financial aid to families, by tweaking the tax code.

Speaking of Canada, there is one recreation centre in particular, in Calgary, Alberta, that has been breaking new ground with kids and fitness. I have worked out at the Westside Recreation Centre and seen the programs offered. So far, it seems like a win for both the Centre and kids' fitness.

Westside caters to adults and seniors, of course, as such places are wont to do, but it also has baby programs, a cool aquatic park, a youth wellness centre, a hockey arena, a leisure ice arena, gymnasiums, a *skateboard park,* outdoor hard courts, a child-minding centre, an education centre that provides resources, and *homework help* for youth 10–17 years of age, private lessons for children, day camps, personal training and sport-specific training, teen facility features—and, yipes, isn't that enough?

Not quite. The fitness and interactive exer-gaming equipment is the latest. Finally, there are youth nights, Friday drop-in games, youth leadership programs, youth volunteer opportunities, and part-time employment.

All that is great, but we folks must be the source of inspiration, and *inspection*. Huh? Our Job One is, well, a reality check. Take a good hard look in the mirror. Ask yourself: Am I chubby? Then look at the child and ask yourself, is my child chubby, or worse?

Because, with common sense, parents don't need a BMI or any other arithmetical diagnostic tool to know if their kid is overweight. They can take a gander at the gaffer and go by the rule of thumb that a picture is worth a thousand words.

In America, at least, the jury is out as to whether parents are clued in. According to a 2010 study, 84% of American parents believe their kids weigh "just right" for their height, yet statistics show that nearly 1/3 of the kids are overweight or obese.

What *may* be just right, and just *what* the doctor ordered, is for parents to find out more about fitness facilities in their communities, to see what they offer the brood. As Westside in Calgary shows, the changes and choices are blooming and beneficial. Hopefully families can frolic, firm up, and forge their way to healthier, happier futures—with a recreation centre helping where, when, and if it can, along the way. For kids' fitness, that will be the day.

Chapter 52
Sack the backpack—Prevent the attack on kids' backs!

Stop obesity before it starts. Sack the backpack. Your children are under attack—and you planned it. Stuffing lunches, GPS tools, books, and toys into the kids' backpacks will give them sicker spines than the Hunchback of Notre Dame.

For shame.

When you add in school supplies, mittens, mats, moisturizers, kittens (just kidding on that one), the whole enchilada can weigh in at up to 3 kilograms (6.61 pounds).

Three kilos is no big deal to adults, but to a 7-year-old tyke, coming in dripping wet at 21 kilos—that's well over 10% of body weight.

What's to be done? While most North American pre-college education is lousy—given the gazillions of gobs of greenbacks to "learn the youngsters" gobbled up—quitting school is not an option. Okay, there is homeschooling. No need for a backpack—and kids do thrive in that environment, though education bureaucrats and teacher unions hate that success and loathe the competition.

Teachers could help by assigning less heavy texts to carry to-and-fro for homework. Betcha the kids would bite on that…

And, while we are here, they'd positively love it if the typical bitching, brawling, Bickerson family did not hitch all the parental pending or post-divorce baggage onto the waif's slender shoulders: they've already got enough weight to tote around without your bad business.

Some parents are badly scared by the possibility that the backpack burden could give kids scoliosis. That, experts generally conclude, is not probable—but sore neck, shoulder, and back muscles are possible—as is rounding of the shoulders, muscles spasms, and distortion of the natural curves of the middle and lower backs—and headaches. So your child is not likely to end up looking like Quasimodo, but something is bound to go wrong if the backpack is so heavy that the kid could tip.

That's the tipping point: Kids off balance fall—and get pranged up that way.

Here are some suggestions to buy the safest (though not necessarily the coolest) backpack.

Make sure it has two straps, not one.

One strap will put undue—and unnecessary strain—on the shoulder or side. You don't want a leaning tower of pipsqueak do you? And if you want an abrasion- and dent-free kid, make sure the shoulder padding is thick enough to prevent ruts from forming. And really, you should think about wheels. If the school says okay, they would really help take a load off ... But if it snows—move to a new warm- climate school scene.

Keep the straps snug and encourage the kid to use the waist strap if the backpack has one.

In the long term, poor posture looms. In the short term: Make room in those emergency rooms. The U.S. saw backpacks causing 7,300 emergency room visits in 2006 (*CNN Health,* September 10, 2007).

Did you know there is a mean—not too lean—American machine overseeing that mean backpack age? Huh? There's no way to properly introduce this...thing, so: It is called the National Electronic Injury Surveillance System (NEISS) of the US Consumer Product Safety Commission (CPSC) National Injury Information Clearinghouse data on backpacks (noted in "Acute backpack injuries in children," *Pediatrics.* 2003 Jan;111(1):163-6).

The mean age of injured kids was 11.8 years. What? Aren't kids meanies from 2 to 20? No, what 11.8 means is that kids between 6 and 18 years old, who reported backpack injuries, averaged out to 11.8...

And gender was neither boon nor barrier: 50% were male.

Oddly enough, back injuries from backpacks ranked as only the 6th most common cause of injury at 11%. The head/face (22%) came first—maybe because brats were brandishing backpacks, swinging them to swat fellow-people pests.

Backpacks attack from all quarters. *Tripping over* these hulky bulks accounted for 28% of the injuries. (And yes, getting clobbered by a backpack added up to an unlucky 13%.)

The Consumer Product Safety Commission (CPSC) said that 89% of backpack injuries *did not* involve the back. Take that—you opening paragraph of shame- less scare-mongering.

And talk about the herd mentality skewing scientific research. Another study found a whopping 97% of kids topped themselves off with a backpack ("Back pain and backpacks in school children," *Journal of Pediatric Orthopedics,* May–June, 2006). Because of their scarcity, kids not toting backpacks couldn't be used as a control group. While that may irk the pointy heads, here is what should bug us: Until Steve Jobs comes back to life to make an iPad/iPod lightweight backpack that can store stuff from attic to dungeon, backpacks are here to stay. The problem is not going away. So what did the *Pediatric Orthopedics* analysis have to say?

Out of 1,540 kids, 37% reported back pain. Of course kids will say anything and some may have told the questioner what he wanted to hear—so hopefully a "fudge factor" was applied. But the use of one or two straps *did not* make an appreciable detrimental or beneficial difference.

Nevertheless, having a three-armed kid—with three straps—next time could spread the risk and the load even more. Better to be safe than sorry. Come to think of it, the kid will be unmercifully bullied—so forget that.

Back to the study. It concluded that school locker availability and a lighter load did have a bearing on back pain.

Backpacks, despite their burdens, are a blessing. They have compartments allowing a child to separate tasks into the "not until hell freezes over" packet, the "over my dead body" pocket, and the "once in a blue moon" pouch.

The rest of life's cr_p can be unceremoniously dumped into the catchall big sack. But the way backpacks are growing, that kid—and backpack—could morph into a *whompus* on campus.

There may be hope for the tykes. High schools such as New York State's, Archbishop Stepinac, are replacing tons of texts with digital versions, stored in an internet "cloud." This trend could filter down to the lower grades.

Chapter 53
LA County Beach ban on football and Frisbee? Geez

One risk we all run increasingly is reduced fitness opportunities due to misplaced concern ...

Los Angeles County has a bounty on your balls and discs.

The County has seen the devil and it is themselves. Only a sinister, sick, evil creature could ban football, Frisbees, and deep-sand digging on public beaches.

Los Angeles County, Los Angeles, and California are beset with astronomical debt disasters, vicious gang warfare, lousy government logistics, businesses leaving, illegal aliens coming, and the last thing the county, city, or state needs to do is kiss off tourism dollars specifically, or fun generally.

This obsession with safety and security is going to kill the aforesaid tourist industry and strangle the ingenuity and inventiveness that used to be the hallmarks of California society. California is regulating itself out of a worthwhile existence, and a recent 37-page ordinance epitomizes the suffocating rot of legislatures that cross every T and dot every I in citizens'—and visitors'—Tom, Dick, and Harry lives.

What's the point of living in the Golden State if living isn't really allowed there?

California dreamin' will be replaced by California scheming as those on the outs of society plot and plan pigskin pitch on the beach. To be fair, they'll be able to engage in toss when the weather is lousier and crowds are down. But between Memorial Day and Labor Day they will be able to throw nothing more than tresses or a tantrum.

Oh, okay, a beach ball or volleyball is hunky dory? Party on! But Fido can't catch a volleyball or beach ball. And this war on frivolity occupies LA County's *70 miles of beaches*? Movin' on to Oregon! Do you hear that drying up of an estimated 50 to 70 million tourists and their bucks?

And they've even put their strong-arm, stupid-head legislative hand in the sand. Unless you are a movie or TV production outfit, don't even think of digging deeper than 18 inches down, otherwise you'll be in deep you-know-what. LA County is worried you might get injured on the beach, in the soft sand. Because they've so minimized hair-raising traffic, road rage, and ghetto rampages, they have nothing else to be concerned about.

Frankly these aren't LA County's biggest problems. On the LA County Web site, under *Crime Information & Prevention,* the map of hot spots looks like barf, that is to say, it's a mess.

A pull-down list uncovers the bad things they haven't competently covered. There's that perennial bugbear of domestic abuse. There's fraud and identity theft. There's substance abuse. So, thank god, they've prioritized and regulated revolving, plastic disks out of site, sight, and mind…

Oops, spoke too soon. It seems this whole brouhaha is nothing more than a tempest in a tea pot. Instead of becoming a dictatorial, bitchy beach society, LA County later *relaxed* the rules of shore play somewhat, rather than tightening them further.

So said LA County officials. But not before they blamed the public for being dense. Except they stated it in a nicer way, cooing that the rule changes had been "badly misunderstood."

Zev Yaroslavsky, the Los Angeles County Supervisor, huffed that this crazy do-not/do stuff has been ruling the waves and lands in the county since 1970. (And for 40 years awareness, acceptance, and accommodation have been misunderstood.)

It seemed that, for whatever reason, international reaction had been due to a misconception. LA County, for 15 minutes of infamy, became a laughing stock. There is *not* a $1,000 fine for a first offense. (That big "G" offense is only if you take off more than your G-string and cavort around naked.) So the fine for bad balls is $100 for a first infraction, and $500 maximum if you goof up three times in one year.

And now, instead of being banned all year round, the offending balls and Frisbees are only out of season during the mid-spring to late summer. And if a lifeguard takes a cotton to you, and you are as sweet as peaches and cream, that overseer may allow you to heave these near-taboo projectiles in designated areas. (No word if reverse-spin Frisbee throws or long-bomb football passes will be allowed.)

It must be grand to have the time to tweak and squeak age-old laws. The luxury of Frisbee or football frolics as your biggest felony to fret about sounds like a lap of living we'd all like to sit on.

Then again, maybe not. The trend towards paternalism in all of Western society, where the god of safety is exalted over the common man's common sense, is becoming a real drag for all but the bureaucrat. Bureaucracies and legislatures are massive monsters run by little people with teeny, terrible minds.

Infantilism is the birthmark of today's digital triple-form typesetting tyrants.

But for now at least, it appears that LA County has taken a step back from the brink. They might not be considered total dinks forever more. And any way you toss it, this ordinance, which actually reduces meddlesomeness, can't be all bad. Play ball!

Chapter 54
Occupy Recess! Toronto school bans balls

(This was written in late 2011. Some players have changed. Dalton McGuinty is no longer premier of Ontario, for one. No loss, he never had balls to begin with.)

Toronto needs some balls. Or at least one school there does. What is going on with the city that frivolity and frolic forgot? First a Toronto ski hill, Centennial Park Ski and Snowboard Centre, banned tobogganing in February 2011, under pressure from the City of Toronto. Now Toronto schools are banning balls? Where does "T.O." get off?

In particular, where does an elementary school, Earl Beatty, get off, with this rather non-ballsy position of banning hard balls? It is being "proactive" says Anna Caputo, Toronto District School Board communications officer. Proactive in cutting down the active.

Are kids destined for birdcages or museums? Will kids' restlessness and resultant pent-up anger put besieged parents in funny farms?

How on earth can children learn to experiment with objects, test their limits, practice skills, improve dexterity, and interact with others in games if balls, a staple of most games, are prohibited? If this trend towards sterile safety continues throughout Toronto—and balls are banned everywhere—kids will never be able to pick up professional sports that demand balls. (Although outside of the Toronto Argonauts who took the 2012 Grey Cup, the other ball teams, the Toronto Raptors, and Blue Jays, have been lousy to mediocre these past few years—so possibly ball playing as a kid doesn't help in ball sports as an adult...)

Anyway. The mentality to cushion us all from life's little bumps and bruises and to protect us from ourselves not only reeks of Big Brother, it peaks as a sorry-sister means to eradicate life experiences. Governments are already banning sugar and salt where they can. So eating fun stuff is becoming taboo—but to administer the boot to the ball right out of kids' lives is stupid and sinister: it's a big booboo.

Balls are round, not sharp. And it's not like youngsters are tossing firecrackers or throwing darts. Yes, true, balls bounce, but that is an advantage—it's hard to play with a no-ricochet pancake. And think of the back injuries that would come with scooping to pick the flat patty up. That wouldn't do.

If I were a rebel kid who was also a bit of a browner, I'd lawyer up, organize a class-action suit, and take the principal, school, school board, and provincial education ministry to court for all they are worth. Which isn't much. The province is flat broke. But, like Greece and California, it deficit spends like crazy, so cash could be had.

What would be the alternative to a world without balls in Toronto, Ontario? Oh—wait—we already know! The province of Ontario, back in 2010, tried to update the kids on ballsy sex. Masturbation would have been taught in Grade 6. The parents went rightfully nuts and the Premier yanked the updated sex education curriculum back to the drawing board (*CBC News*, April 22, 2010).

Dalton McGuinty was that Ontario Premier. He was known as "Premier Dad." Mostly derisively. He is a complete wuss, a patsy who couldn't say no to any union demand, no matter how pricey. But in this case he did say no, or at least passed the buck (even though he's the provincial boss) saying Earl Beatty Public School's ball ban was... worthy of further dialog.

Couldn't he just say they were complete fools? He tried a joke: Balls aren't registered weapons. Is that the best he could do? Then he said something serious that was dumber than his limp laugh line. He said he wanted kids to be active and safe—but everybody knows the two don't always go together. If one can't toss a ball or shush down a hill, the safety factor is super but the activity factor stinks. (Unless, that is, the kids give those eyeball muscles a workout, in envy and from afar, watching kids in other jurisdictions doing kid stuff.)

The Earl Beatty Public School Web site welcomes visitors in a zillion languages—so long as they don't have balls. They now say the ball ban is temporary; in reality, it will probably stay in place until nobody gets hurt by a ball anywhere, physically and geographically.

There is hope. Ten-year-old Mathew Taylor faced a ball ban at Lockview elementary school in St. Catharines, Ontario (*St. Catharines Standard*, November 7, 2011). He rustled up 94 other petitioners, met with Principal Candy McMillan, and convinced her to reverse the perverse ban. He said the kids were tired of standing around doing nothing during recess.

Speaking of zillions, big talk radio host Rush Limbaugh lambasted the ban, saying this *wimpify* process would turn tykes into wusses. *Saturday Night Live* also lampooned the dumbness.

But it is no laughing matter. Certainly the 100 or so protesting kids yelling "We want our balls back!" (*Toronto Star*, November 16, 2011) didn't think so. Occupy Recess is the battle cry! Many schools have already stomped out, or put these activities/equipment on the endangered list: tag, red rover, see-saws, snowball fights... Is all this right?

So soccer's scrapped. Detractors may snipe, so what? Canada, except for the ladies' 2012 Olympic team, generally sucks at soccer anyway, so what's the big deal? But things could change, if that ball were not verboten. Let's say a kid has no experience with balls until he becomes an adult. And then by a fluke of nature he's hit by one. Will a complaint be made to the UN Office on Disarmament Affairs?

Perhaps not too surprisingly, the Earl Beatty school blurb omits talking about children's physical development: "Our teachers are dedicated to continuous professional learning and we are committed to providing a balanced curriculum which addresses the *personal, social and academic needs of our children.*"

Oh, the nerds have since decreed Nerf balls to be okay. And to think that it all happened just because *one adult* got a concussion from getting beaned by a ball. Heave ho—the volleyballs, tennis balls, footballs and therefore about *350 kids'* fun in recreation all had to go.

Gotta blow for the kids huh? And suck.

Chapter 55

Quebec's "Weight Coalition" wants to ban and tax soft drinks

Governments declare war on obesity, smoking
Here...

Should a Quebec-based group "Weight Coalition" single out soda pop punitive taxation in the battle against obesity and weight gain? They proposed this measure back on February 3rd, 2011, and a peek at their Web site in 2013 shows that they're still at it.

Silly or scrupulous? According to the beverage industry association, such a tax, far from being logical, is ludicrous. Representatives of the sugar industry also said there is no conclusive evidence to tie obesity directly to soft drinks. Statistics Canada reports that consumption of soft drinks has actually decreased over the last decade, while obesity rates continue to rise. Not that this deters the Weight Coalition. Frankly, they sound like heavyweight busybodies, sticking their noses into our business. None of their concerns address the real factors driving obesity and weight gain: personal choice and lack of individual initiative. The idea behind the "soda tax" is that the taxes collected, say an extra one cent per litre, will be used to fight obesity. The funds will not go directly to fat folks, however; they will be swallowed up by government, starting new programs to stem the spike in spongy, soft bodies.

The Canadian government already has an organization called Participaction. One of its slogans aimed at getting mushy Canadians to move is, more or less, a taunt: "Dare 2 Move." Participaction talks of the "inactivity crisis." Participaction, judging by its board members, has been incredibly successful, but not so much in averting this inactivity crisis, but rather in declaring itself worthy and wonderful. It declares—raves—that Participaction itself is an iconic brand. Granted, it isn't soda pop, but maybe, as a brand, it could be taxed. And the monies leached thereby could be used to fight obesity…

The Weight Coalition and other NGO or government nosenheimers should cut us all some slack. Unpleasant though it may be, if folks want to waste time idly watching their waists grow, isn't that *their* beeswax? Concerned types say no, it is everybody's business because the obese are a drain on the public purse, blah, blah, blah. Haw. Obese people die sooner—as a result, they hardly impact the boomer aging crisis, with its attendant medical bills. And let's face it; this well-meaning, best-of-intentions initiative to single out and pick on pop, as our source of liquid refreshment, is essentially grubby people grasping at straws. You and I should grasp our love handles and take control of our own weight problems, if only to curb the voracious appetites of associations and organizations seeking to meddle in our bulging, bungled affairs.

These associations and organizations, culminating or collapsing with the omnibus of government bureaucracy, are funny. Not funny, tee-hee, but funny the way they view and term life. A quick glance at obesity rates in Canada took me to Wikipedia. There, emblazoned in the first sentence is this daunting declaration: "Obesity in Canada … is one of the leading causes of preventable deaths in Canada." This is dumb. There is, to date, no such thing as a preventable death in Canada or anywhere else, as death is determined to destroy life, 100% of the time. Maybe they should have said early death. Or maybe they should perish that thought. Better yet, perish as an official entity.

With respect to Quebec, a study in 2004 titled "Canadian Community Health Survey" (and even here, whoever scrawled this title could lose 25% of its excess baggage just by calling it "Canadian Health Survey") had Quebec near the bottom, 2nd best. In other words, Quebec had near the lowest percentages of obese and overweight citizenry. From 2004 to 2009, researchers say, the numbers of Quebec fatties remained largely unchanged, nestling in between 20% and 24%. And, as the obesity maps prepared by a team at the University of British Columbia's School of Population and Public Health show, Quebec's obesity rates *have risen* since 2010 to 25% to 29%. But that still leaves them firmly in the middle of the provincial and territorial fat pack. (Betcha the Weight Coalition will use these facts as adipose ammunition to butt into all Canadians' lives…)

Back to our "soda pop" tax. This is but one of the Weight Coalition's big plans. Another is a ban on the sale of soft drinks and energy drinks in federal buildings across Canada. Suzie Pellerin, President of the organization, says that that is a reality already in many public buildings in Quebec.

Pellerin has to know that the Quebec government bureaucracies lead the way in Canada in promoting huge, fat, corpulent numbers of government employees. If she wants governments to lead by example, she could advocate that they cut the fat in staffing, and leave us the pleasure of an occasional soft drink without viciously clubbing us via a one cent per litre excise tax.

The Coalition claims, on its Web site, that counteracting obesity is a collective challenge. It is not. It is up to the individual. I can hector you to lose lard and you can lecture me to mind my own backyard. No one adult can make another adult lose weight (let us leave kids out of this for now, shall we?), whether through the carrot or stick. Another of the Coalition's aims is to target food marketers. Apparently if too many of us find out that food is available we may go off the deep end and eat the stuff. Presumably, they want to investigate and regulate advertisements and the claims they make. But that is not what their little blurb says: it just says, target food marketing.

At the very most, governments, rather than negatively sanctioning food and drink deemed evil, should positively sanctify food and drink deemed heavenly. The Canadian government has had its collective arm twisted, for instance, to make healthy foods less expensive through tax reform. But whether governments, associations, or organizations are pro or con on certain foods—and wish to push their views on the masses— they imply that we, the lorded over and lambasted, are too dumb to know what we should or should not eat and drink.

Chapter 56
Nathan's Hot Dog Eating Contest 2011

Although this piece was written a couple of years back, some things never change. Joey Chestnut won The 2013 Nathan's Hot Dog Eating contest, wolfing back 69 hot dogs in ten minutes. It was his seventh win in a row. Now on with the goings on in the 2011 show!

Nathan's Hot Dog Eating Contest—is this some kind of hellish, coquettish, fetish with hot dogs we relish—or what? This gastronomical game, where first place wins $10,000, exudes Epicureanism at its eeriest and easiest. It's gotta be simple, right, for who'd gobble, shovel, and swallow tens of hotdogs in 10 minutes if it wasn't a breeze…

Try it, you'll gag.

Joey "Jaws" Chestnut sure doesn't. He certainly has *the* stomach for hovering over hotdogs, is a tough nut to crack, and won his fifth consecutive Nathan's Hot Dog Eating Contest on July 4th, 2011, on Coney Island, New York. The native Californian stands tall in this "sport." He is six feet tall and, surprisingly, pretty thin, considering his pastime (career, avocation, obsession, hobby, odd job, if you like); he comes in at about 218 pounds. Add around five more pounds in weight, after he polishes off 60-plus buns and wieners.

Every Superman needs a Lex Luthor. Unfortunately, Takeru "Tsunami" Kobayashi, the Japanese main-man threat to the Chestnut, was ineligible for this year's meet n' eat of meat. He was, however, eligible for a night in jail in 2010, after being charged with disorderly conduct when he clambered up on the stage "in the heat of it." Tough stuff.

Aside from Mr. Kobayashi's "staged" dispute, how could *anyone* be declared ineligible for the desire and dedication to stuff himself silly for the greater girth of mankind?

Mankind now includes women too. This year, the first Women's Hot Dog Eating Contest was won by a new number one, Sonya Thomas, aka "The Black Widow."

But Joey Chestnut, seen holding a big pink bottle of Pepto Bismol while interviewed, is in a class by himself. He wolfed 62 dogs down, a full nine more than second place's Pat Bertoletti, who downed eight more than third place finisher Tim Janus, who mustered 45.

Certainly ESPN, which televised the contest, treated it like a sport, breathlessly remarking how Joey started munching at a "blistering, record-setting pace." Joey, with his stock clichés like "I did what I had to do," helped give the spectacle a professional impression. And the mustard yellow championship belt doesn't hurt...

Big debate. Does Joey Chestnut rate? As an athlete? ESPN's Skip Bayless emphatically says yes, pointing out that Joey must have super breathing control and cardio capabilities, so he won't literally choke on the job, and he notes that Joey is "pretty ripped."

Joey would probably have a rip-roaring good time with Don Gorske. The latter has a Big Mac love-a-thon going. He's eaten over 25,000 in his lifetime, but he's a marathon man, not a sprinting gullet shoveler like Joey is.

Suppose you are not a leaner towards the wiener. No problemo. There are lots of competitions for other comestibles you can sink your teeth into: pepperoni rolls, oysters, Buffalo chicken wings, and baby back ribs, to name a few.

1.677 is under a few. Sorry, that's 1.677 *million*, that's how many people watched the 2010 Hot Dog spectacle live, courtesy of ESPN, with another 40,000 or so souls on hand. ESPN had the rights to this year's 96th show and has, in fact, had the exclusive rights to coverage since 2004.

We could chew the fat over hot dogs, but, after all, we know what they are. And we're sure making them, is icky. But what is IFOCE? It is "The International Federation of Competitive Eating."

Isn't a regulatory agency for a binge a little hard to stomach? Can't folks simply unwind, forcing hot dogs into their system, without Big Brother getting his knickers in a knot?

Er, no. The stakes are high. Tension prevails. Ten minutes is all you have to prove your mettle. Should you, ahem, have a "reversal of fortune," you are disqualified. If you spill, spew, and splatter too much hot dog, you may be issued a yellow card.

And no one can sally up on the stage for this, *the* prestigious event of hot dog downing, unannounced. Qualifying contests are held to weed out weak eaters, mere pretenders.

Have the champions, with a title to defend, a "force" with them? Yes—they have elastic stomachs, trained and tutored in stretching capacity, conditioned by drinking scads of water while in training.

Back to IFOCE. It extols an outfit called Major League Eating on its Web site. Can you guess who they are? No, really, this is literally the world—no pun intended—body (MLE) that holds and oversees about 80 events per year. We are told that "MLE promotions generate more than a billion consumer impressions worldwide each year."

Understated that, consumer impressions...

It's impossible to avoid the impression that Joey Chestnut has his finger in many pies. He's voluminously versatile; he demolished over nine pounds of deep fried asparagus spears at the Stockton Asparagus Fest this past April.

The health and medical industries certainly aren't awed. They are, in fact, aghast that such fast-food feasts/fests live and thrive. They feel gluttony is lionized and reckon that viewers watching Joey eat a million of whatever is at stake, piled in front of him that day, might ignore uncontrolled portion sizes and risk obesity.

While the contrast between this not-so-sumptuous repast and starvation in the Horn of Africa is ghastly, seen by itself it is just a celebration, albeit a weird and wacky one, of the freedoms extant in the USA. Independence Day, July 4th, and Nathan's Hot Dog Eating Contest have been linked like old-fashioned frankfurters for decades. Unlike the temporarily terribly bloated stomachs of the fun food warriors, the tradition shows no signs of diminishing. Wouldn't it be wonderful if all the "action" was on the battlefield of the buffet, with a side order of a "Takeru temper" tempura thrown in?

No sin there.

Chapter 57
Mayor Bloomberg's Soda Ban

There...

Bill de Blasio became the New York mayor on January 1st, 2014. And he may turn out to be even more of a busybody than the outgoing bossy Bloomberg.

Why is elected New York mayor and self-appointed public nanny Michael Bloomberg so freaked out over the people's fannies? Has New York no municipal issues that could otherwise occupy his time? Or is he just a know-it-all who simply can't resist making New Yorkers stop drinking sodas in sizes he can't stomach?

Bloomberg's pestering has a lot of backfield support. The New York City Department of Health and Mental Hygiene, led by Health Commissioner Thomas Farley, a natural ally, has 6,000 employees and a $1.6 billion budget all a-hum to fix the bum. Farley and Bloomberg make a powerful tag team, a one-two punch ramming all sorts of health mandates at the people. Overbearing? For sure. Overzealous? Could be.

Journalist Lowen Liu ("All Hail the Nanny State," *Slate*, Oct. 23, 2012) would disagree with the "overbearing, overzealous" rap. He makes a pretty compelling case for Mayor Bloomberg's ban on sodas larger than 16 ounces at restaurants and concessions. Liu likes the Bloomberg's approach. He sees it as incremental, tolerable, doable.

He also points to some incredible statistics. Since 1990, when New Yorkers lived three years less than the average American, their life expectancy rates have exploded, tacking on *eight years,* as compared to the comparatively paltry 1.7 years per decade other Americans added on.

Why the huge uptick? Less "... heart disease, cancer, diabetes, and stroke."

(Whether having New Yorkers live longer is beneficial, is best left for history to decide.)

And, besides his tactics, Bloomberg has another thing in his favor, his acumen. Set aside, for a moment, the annoying accent, the pretentiousness of his apparent belief that people will listen to a civic politician, and his pettiness in arbitrarily mandating that anything larger than one 16-ounce size is a stop-the-show, no-go flow. You have to admire his prescience in knowing there's no way his voters will figure out a workaround like ordering, say, two 16-ounce sized drinks. Not gonna happen.

Actually, the Boston-born Bloomberg has pretty much been a huge success all his life, starting from his schooling at Johns Hopkins University and Harvard Business School to his IT work at Salomon Brothers to his starting up a company called Bloomberg LP, to his charity work, so it's no wonder he knew he'd be persuasive with his soda ban. Maybe Bloomberg should take his act statewide. At that level an estimated one third, or 1.4 million kids are obese or overweight. For sure, New York big-bean counter, State Comptroller Thomas P. DiNapoli, would welcome his bossy ways with open arms. DiNapoli is trying to get his head around the havoc obesity rates are wrecking by voraciously gobbling up a greater and greater slice of the state spending pie. Yet DiNapoli should give his head a shake. His prescription of what must be done is all smoke and mirrors, a pipe dream, a hookah. He invites everybody and anybody from a grab bag of disparate groups, more familiar with infighting than uniting, to tie one on in order to put a metaphorical tourniquet on rampant tubbiness: "We—educational agencies, health departments, medical providers, community organizations, families, elected officials, the media, religious groups, and all concerned citizens—must work together expeditiously to reduce the human and financial costs of obesity on all New Yorkers."

That'll be the day.

If Bloomberg's soda ban doesn't lose its fizz and DiNapoli's got the chops for it, they both might want to check out New Yorkers' wombs, because that is where the obesity egg is laid. Or so say researchers at the Charite Hospital of Berlin, who analyzed 640,000 births across 26 countries. They concluded that an infant who weighed over 4 kg at birth had twice the chance of adult obesity (*Times of India*, February 11, 2013). Oh my, the two hassling handwringers can groan and deliver sermons on slimness while moms moan and deliver small fry suitably sized for New York State.

If Bloomberg ever tires of pushing, poking, and prodding New Yorkers this way and that, he might want to move to California where a new field poll shows that the majority of Californians support a tax on sugary drinks, so long as the funds are then spent on anti-obesity programs and physical education.

Or, better still, mayor Michael might make Manhattan move to the mountain because, brainiac maniac that he is, he has got to be aware that the higher the home altitude, the thinner the air, and the less obesity (*Reuters Health*, February 12, 2013).

Clearly, a miracle man's work is never done. Or as Bloomberg blurts: "We're simply forcing you to understand…" Actually, this year, the ban was struck down by a court and is now winding its way through the court of appeals. On a personal note, I am shocked that a municipal government thinks that such bans are any of its business. You'd think the city was an elementary school cafeteria.

Perhaps Mayor Bloomberg should understand this. Before he goes absolutely off the deep end and attacks big rear ends with a fat tax, Denmark can say, been there, done that—and the whole thing fell flat.

It didn't work out too well. Except for Germany. They did not have *fedtafgiften*, a fat tax. So when Danish mandarins started taxing cheese and milk, and, believe it or not, dried apricots coated in oily wax paper, Danes scampered over to Germany to buy from German businesses that were only too happy to proclaim that they did not have to charge tax on fatty foods.

Denmark's fat tax, the *world's first*, died a pretty quick death. It was born 2011 and was beheaded in 2012 (*The Economist*, November 17, 2012).

Chapter 58
Los Angeles City Council forbids fast food

The Los Angeles City Council has, as of December 2010, forbidden new fast food outlets from opening in south LA. What they have obtusely and crazily ordained reflects the overseer mentality of omnipotence, dictating what residents may, or may not, eat. As councilman Bernard Parks barks: "...We don't think our community needs to have 10 or 15 or 18 ways to eat a hamburger."

Why not? Who is this councilman to judge what fast food suits or doesn't suit those who choose to chomp around? Doesn't Los Angeles have more pressing concerns than the size of its constituents—like, according to the LAPD—the estimated 400 gangs that roam freely? Are not individuals, there and throughout the USA, constitutionally gifted with the right to life, liberty, and the pursuit of happiness even if their pants and dresses don't fit quite right? Obesity rates in south LA have ramped up Los Angeles City Council to run roughshod over prospective businesses via regulation. This is meddling—by peddling that Papa LA Council knows best.

What is the point of living if you can't live large and go hell-bent-for-leather, gulping juicy onion-and-mushroom-slathered half-pounder hamburgers, topped off by chocolate fudge ice cream sundaes? Surely citizens, in south LA and throughout LA, are excused if they go off the deep end in frustration and anger, watching politicians fiddle and diddle while south LA sinks into slums. And who is this Los Angeles council to point its busybody fingers at its citizenry anyway? Since the 1990s, through the usual noxious political chicanery, this council has, by means of fine print within "Measure H," enjoyed automatic raises. Every time municipal judges got a raise, they did too. This obscenity is far more grievous than perceived or pronounced obesity.

The average annual take-home pay for these very average men and women, who do a below average job, is now some $178,000. These financial fat cats should be glad their denizens don't turn to alcohol to blow off steam, and sink the council into its chambers. If the common ruck ever wakes up—then the council would be in the muck and have a real big problem to ponder about.

It is easy to fathom why the Los Angeles council frets and sweats about concerns on the far edges of its mandate. Instead of cleaning up their own sordid swamp, they can take swipes at John Doe and Suzy Q, who simply choose to dine out at a fast food venue.

This is another example of government targeting legal businesses while doing nothing about, say, those hundreds of unruly gangs. And when the LAPD states that violent crime is down 3.9%, let us take that with a grain of salt. For example, we were told that rapes decreased 5 whole percent for the four-week period ending January 15th, 2011, from the earlier four-week period ending December 18th, 2010! If we put it in numerical terms, 19 persons were raped this latest period instead of the 20 raped the period previous. Big advance. Los Angeles has many vexations and vices: obesity isn't at the top of the heap.

Besides, why on earth does a municipal government care a whit about fatties in the first place? Which body politic is constitutionally responsible for health concerns? The states and the feds. And the feds, with Obamacare, would now seem to already have a monopoly on intrusiveness. Municipal governments, well meaning or otherwise, should stick to their knitting. And if they don't know what that knitting is, maybe somebody can pass them the Los Angeles City Charter. There, under "Rules & Policies," electricity, water, and trees are the points of concern. Stuff that affects streets. Basics. Essentials. Integrals. Menu choices behind restaurant or fast food joint doors are peripherals and should be nobody's business, save the server's and the eater's.

Good intentions, too, are undoubtedly behind the nixing of new fast food establishments in south LA. One can almost hear the hand wringers now: Don't you know we mean well? And know all? If it weren't for us, you might live lives of individuality and initiative. Free to make your own choices. Free to screw up by pigging out. This way you can relax, though not in a fast food joint. Chill, knowing we are warm to your form, cocooning you with protection from such mayhem as personal cuisine preferences. Your basic needs like food are our responsibility. But, ahem, uh, well, oh, by the way—the "Los Angeles Budget Challenge," launched January 27th, lets you—that same citizen—well let us read their exact words...

The Los Angeles Budget Challenge is an interactive online tool that lets you solve the City's budget deficit...

Because we, the LA Council, are unable or unwilling to do so, being up in arms about how much fast food you are eating.

A July 2003 report titled: "LAHEALTH—Obesity on the Rise" paints a pretty ugly picture of how LA County citizens look and waddle. They break the statistics down by race, with African Americans the greatest weight "offenders," followed by Latino Americans, then Whites, then Asians.

The obesity rate in 2002 was highest among African-Americans (31%), followed by Latinos (24%), Whites (16%), and Asians (6%) (Figure 1). The obesity rate was also higher among those with less education and low household incomes...

There is no reason to assume that the numbers haven't worsened. In fact, if we are to believe bureaucracies like the World Health Organization (WHO), the number and percentage of obese people everywhere has worsened considerably, and right now, unfortunately, those folks are ahead of me in the buffet line.

You know what? If we can't eat what we want, and do, therefore, break some pending or current municipal by-law or regulation, will the punishment be a revocation of toilet privileges? Look, we know cigarettes are not life-sustaining and neither is alcohol, though you might get an argument on the latter from writers. But food is; and whether the Los Angeles councilors like it or not, we can survive, if not thrive, on junk food. And if folks burn more calories than they consume through fat food, and healthy food, there is even less of a "problem" not to worry about. If these fussy food-o-crats from LA want to live our lives, let them go whole hog and ensure that we get salaries like theirs, with automatic pay raises. Otherwise don't let the door hit your fat ass on the way out.

Chapter 59
British obesity—money for the massive

The British Labour government has laboured over the idea of paying its fat citizens. They would get money, vouchers, or other rewards just because they were overweight. The only catch is, they had to shed this weight, to come down to a "healthy weight." This idea was tossed around in 2007– 2008 and was then announced by Health Secretary Alan Johnson.

Back then, nearly a quarter of British adults were obese and nearly a fifth of children were. A 2010 Health Survey for England (HSE) reported that 26.1% of adults were obese, along with 16% of kids. So the adults were up a percentage point, while many youngsters may or may not have lost weight—it depends on what the 2007 definition of "nearly a fifth of children" means exactly.

While the meaning of the figures was still under discussion, the government shoveled aside 372 million pounds for a pay-for-weight-loss strategy. Alan Johnson, the Health Secretary, and Ed Balls, the Secretary of State for Children, Schools and Families, hoped that England would become "the first leading nation to reverse the trend for expanding waistlines, especially among children." (*Politics Forum*, January 24, 2008).

The term "healthy weight" was not defined in the article but let's hope that the government did not plan an oh-so-easy, sleazy, slimeball move to change the healthy weight definition(s) just as folks were within reach. Or, to justify further meddling.

There were to have been annual reports charting the progress. Bureaucrats, more than likely, snooping around, ferreting out the fat, would themselves have gotten thinner. So the suit spies would have directly benefited even if they were despised by your bulky, basic-giant Jane and her wide sidekick, gargantuan Joe.

Here's how the government planned to be a pain in the ass: It wanted to pester parents, though they use the gentler word, persuade, to stop feeding their kids bad food. They wanted to use 30 million pounds to create "healthy towns," which should have pissed off every British county, borough, district, and unitary authority. They wanted compulsory cooking lessons in schools, which should have provoked food fights, especially if people are peeved about pork. They wanted "walking buses" where adults would walk kids to school, which should have put perverts on high alert. They wanted parents to spy on kids' computer time, which should have induced a swill of ill will as soon as the computer savvy offspring found out what their folks had been up to. They wanted a "single system for food labeling" which should have riled the job creators (businesses), saddled with unnecessary costs to suit the whim rule of the day.

Why this pie-in-the-sky try—to fritter away cash on the big fat fans of the fantastic french fry (chips)?

Well, we were told,

Obesity is linked to an increased risk of cancer, heart and liver disease and diabetes... It is predicted that 60 per cent of men, 50 per cent of women and 25 per cent of children could be obese by 2050 if action is not taken.

Alan Johnson, the Health Secretary for the government said: "The core of the problem is simple—we eat too much and we do too little exercise. The solution is more complex."

Raise the red flag. If the core of the problem was simple, why was the answer not simple too? Why is the solution complex? Was it to justify further governmental oversight into our lives? For sure, governmental regulation and bureaucratic strangulation would propagate themselves, in the fertile soil of new powers and responsibilities.

The government was not going whole hog into this. It decided to set out with pilot projects before introducing the idea nationally. Essentially, it would be buying off the obese with taxpayer funds. One suspected that the healthy would soon have claimed victim status so as to get their share of the loot.

Fast forward to now. Labour has been out of power in the UK since 2010. A quick glance at the shadow cabinet news stories at their Web site as of January 18th, 2013, shows that for the first three pages they harangue the current government for everything but the kitchen sink, but make no mention of obesity in Britain today. Perhaps the Labour party has lost interest in the rotund...

The current government, the Conservative Party, makes no mention of the money-for-the-massive plan Labour toyed with. Instead, its signature document of October 13th, 2011, is: Healthy Lives, Healthy People: A call to action on obesity in England. It murmurs and muses about "partnerships"—a clear indication that it believes that government can't do it alone.

Here's who they consider their point men: PCT CEs, NHS Trust CEs, SHA CEs, Care Trust CEs, Foundation Trust CEs, Medical Directors, Directors of PH, Directors of Nursing, Local Authority CEs, Directors of Adult SSs, PCT Chairs, NHS Trust Board Chairs, Allied Health Professionals, GPs, Communications Leads, and Directors of Children's Social Services.

Even if picking organizations with cryptic names seems odd, the government, intentionally or not, offers a nice play on words with its opening chapter. Chapter 1 is titled: The scale of the challenge.

Anyway, Prime Minister David Cameron's present government means well. They're concerned and caring, and they wear their feelings on their sleeves as they dress down anyone in society who displeases them.

Oh, by the by, did you know there is also a British Obesity Society? And no, it isn't an agglomeration of chubby elite wine swishers who get together to chew the fat. It is a group that strives to be "inclusive" and wants to have as its members "everyone affected by obesity in the UK." Yikes, that should make it the largest deliberative, contemplative body in the whole wide world.

Unlike Alan Johnson, mentioned above, they believe the factors behind obesity involve so much more than lack of exercise and an abundance of chowing down: "… genetics, physiology, biochemistry and the neurosciences, as well as environmental, psychological and cultural factors."

But like Alan Johnson they want the government to be more involved, like yesterday. Obese people upset them and they want them done away with (or at least made skinnier.) They want discipline, or at the minimum a "multidisciplinary effort" to manage the current levels of obesity and to prevent the masses of the great unwashed from getting bigger and bigger, in both senses.

But just because your local obesity society, governments of every stripe and hue, and friends and family bug you to shape up or ship out, you and I won't so much as move a muscle, other than to get out of earshot, if we, deep down in our hearts and with every twitching fiber of our body, don't covet and crave with an intense desire—the goal of losing weight.

Without our own personal initiative, all the king's horses and all the king's men can't put Humpty (Dumpty) together again as a more svelte, shapely, healthy soul.

The proof is in the pudding. Britain has been designated the "fat capital" of Europe, according to a recent study from the University of Madrid's School of Medicine.

Maybe *this* will end up being the only way the British government can think of to help the adipose afflicted: "Fat families are to be prescribed a visit to their local Sainsbury's by GPs, where they will be taken by the hand and shown healthy foods."

Chapter 60
Skinned alive! Paul Mason, World's Fattest Man

The pictures are hard enough to view but the story is even harder to hear. Have you seen the before and after photos of Paul Mason? He weighed a million pounds, lost a ton, and now shows more skin than a professional stripper on perpetual tour.

Congratulations are in order for the British bloke. Losing weight is not easy, even if he resorted to gastric bypass surgery. Officially, he lost 40 stone, or 560 pounds. But now he wants his hard-pressed fellow taxpayers to pitch in so he can get his loose skin surgically removed.

Shouldn't that be his financial responsibility? Just where are the boundaries between personal and public onus these days? You gotta give him credit—the guy once billed as the *World's Fattest Man* has equal parts balls and chutzpah.

As the world's fattest man, he was used to being feted. But he wasn't force fed was he? No one ordered him to become obese, did they? No one, save he, enjoyed the bounteous banquets and the sumptuous repasts, did they?

Paul sure could put it back. He used to chow down some 20,000 calories per day. That works out to 5.71 pounds daily. Take that and multiply it by 365, and by a typical year's end he would have gained, let's see, um, uh, 2,085.71 pounds, except of course, that much of the energy went to maintaining his huge metabolism.

The miracles and mysteries of calorie burn-off must have been at work on Paul, a former postman. And, miracle upon miracle, it's not like he hasn't used the state before to fund his unfathomable ways; he has. The National Health Service (NHS) paid for his gastric bypass. It cost 30,000 British pounds. That's not chicken feed. And two women spend hours daily washing him. That's a pretty good deal. Lots of gents would groove to that. And get this: "His care bill costs taxpayers an estimated £100,000 a year, and it is believed to have topped £1million over the past 15 years." (*Daily Mail,* November 25, 2011).

Paul Mason may be a fine fellow—if not for some strange inconsistencies in his ideas on who should be running his personal ship of state. He wants the NHS and the taxpayer to do this and that, yet reserves the final timing of this proposed excess skin removal surgery to his own whims and wishes.

Reactions range from disgust, dismay, and derision to disbelief. Just kidding, that's just the gamut of feelings that well up and flow out upon rereading Mr. Mason's tale of terrible turmoil. Clearly it is, as they say, all about *him*, and while it may seem normal to him that the world revolve around his being—for that being has occupied his every thought and non-action for years now—it should be apparent to this gentleman that others have an interest—and not just as a source of funding—in his plaintive pleas as well.

Take the NHS. Amazingly, they haven't told Mason to take the proverbial hike. Rather astoundingly, they seem to be looking out for his best interests—even if Paul, myopic and selfish, can't see what those interests are.

Before they consider paying for the piles of skin to be pared off, they want to make sure that the prospective patient's weight has stabilized. Makes sense doesn't it? It's not like this is an order-on-demand pizza service is it? Medical care means that technically trained staff must be available and operations are costly.

Mr. Mason isn't a dough head. Besides his post office skills, he has a knack for crafts: he wants to make birthday cards and Christmas tree decorations. He even had his own TV Show, *Britain's Fattest Man*. He's a self-promoter, albeit in a weird and not-so-wonderful way.

Given that he has a modicum of smarts, why would he blame the NHS for not doing more to help prevent his weight gain in the first place? Surely, he knows he's responsible for what goes into the old pie hole and that to rely on a bureaucracy—even a well meaning one—as a solution to one's problems is fatuous at best and fat-headed at worst.

He's angry that the NHS told him to "ride his bike more." Sounds like sage advice. The fact that he couldn't get up (for about a decade) to get on the bike that he could not even see below the belly rolls—to take that ride—is not their problem.

It's his.

He should be able to figure out that walking might have been a good place to start. It has worked as a weight-reducing technique for zillions of people for eons of ages. It's free. It may not be as sexy as a personalized program with a trainer, but hey, it's better than a kick in the head.

Mr. Mason probably needs a kick in the keester. It might boot into him some initiative to figure out where he can start earning money to pay privately for the skin removal operation pronto, if that is the way he wants to go. Because that's the alternative. (Other than to continue complaining and carping.)

He'll need to fork over anywhere from £1,500 to £6,000 for the procedure. Maybe he can tap a friend or a relative who hasn't disowned him yet, if he's hard up. If he wants this skinning operation like, lickety split, he'll think of something. Every parent knows there are baby cries, and then there are *baby cries*. One learns to distinguish between authentic anguish and an addled, frantic antic.

No doubt the skin hanging here there and everywhere is unsightly. Most of us don't show off our bad parts, even when we are stoned or soused. But in this whale of a story, it seems Paul Mason shares photos willingly. Is this to induce sympathy and raise a little bread, or is he not so disgusted with his rolls as he'd have us believe—and is he thus playing with our collective head?

Oh, here's the latest. Is Rebecca Mountain a head case? She's an American with a sense for ??? and, as of November 2013, has fallen for Paul Mason harder than Obamacare has fallen from grace. She and Paul have set up a shed-the-skin-surgery online fundraising page, their target: 16,000 pounds. And that's for travelling and drugs etc., to the US where a doctor has offered to do the operation for free, or for a song, or for publicity, one might suppose. We're talking eight stone of skin. For those not familiar with stone(s) measurement, try 114 pounds or nearly 51 kilograms. As for Rebecca, she sells cat toys for a living. And now she has a new pet cause to coddle.

The mind boggles.

Chapter 61
Obese 700-pound woman Donna Simpson
wants to be 1000 pounds… maybe…

Donna Simpson is batting a thousand. Or the 700-pound gal will be, if she ever reaches her goal to be "Miss Obesity Universality." Everybody should have a goal, right? Even if the goal is wrong. A Miss Obesity Universality may not even exist, but rest assured, Donna does. Guinness Book of Records, anyone?

She figures 1000 pounds, or a paltry 300 pounds more than she weighs now, ought to do the trick and get her the coveted fat-female-of-the-firmament award. Donna is driven. Donna is determined.

Donna's persuasive too: her four year old daughter is on her side. She also has a 15-year-old son.

Just because someone has a large ass, doesn't preclude them being smart. She reportedly makes $100,000 per year (*Daily Mail,* July 6, 2011).

Scholars, health practitioners, hand-wringers and anyone underneath Donna may have a bone to pick with her and wonder whether "going for the big fat" is a big bad.

Or should we, rather, praise a woman who isn't willing to settle for second best, and isn't willing to let anything stand in her way, except maybe standing up, in her quest to become the World's Most Obese Woman?

Donna's in her early forties and apparently, to meet her mark (and possibly, her maker), must put back some 12,000 to 15,000 calories per day. The exact numbers vary, depending on the article read. Why this or that number? What if she ate, say, a measly 6,000 calories per day? Wouldn't that merely mean she'd take twice the time to reach the round thou?

Hey—on just whose dime is all this dining done? On hers? She forks over $600 to $750 weekly, for food. That's a lot of bread.

Actually, she's a self-made woman in more senses than one. She says she has 7,000 fee-paying fans watching her feed herself.

Oh. Er, um, okay.

So this is all on her nickel. She's earned her money the old fashioned way, not through victimhood or bitching for government entitlements, but by building a, well, bigger mousetrap.

Listen, are you going to argue with her? If she throws her weight around intellectually—as well as she packs it on physically—she's sure to win any debate, hands down.

Speaking of down, who's going to look after the kids when she's not around? How did she get pregnant in the first place? And those attracted to her beefing up—what's that all about—this fat fetish? Feederism is a part of this fetish. No guff. Who makes up this stuff?

More questions gurgle up.

Should we freak that the little daughter might want to grow up to be "just like mommy?" When Donna wants to relax, kick back, take a load off—does she eat less? How does the washroom thing work?

We know some governments have taken kids from their parents if the kids were deemed too fat. Will a government take a parent deemed too fat away from the kids?

How can Donna tell if one of her socks is the wrong color? Who cuts her baby toenails? Are fat jokes okay, now that Donna Simpson is showboating the way?

Is junk food hunky dory for her to eat? Eating healthy is meaningless when one chooses corpulence, correct?

How much time does it take to chow down 12,000 calories? Does eating "fast food" help? Do Jerome Bettis ("The Bus") and William Perry ("The Refrigerator") posters adorn her boudoir walls?

Her man, Robert Simpson, "supports her hobby." Let's hope, not literally. Robert weighs 150 pounds.

And isn't hobby the wrong word? Isn't this vocation, this devotion—of stacking and packing —more of a lifestyle career choice? Who was the high school guidance counselor that helped with this big decision?

She says she's not harming anyone. She also says she loves eating. It's hard not to argue with the first point. It's easy as pie to agree with the second.

Some might say she has an eating disorder. Balderdash. Her eating is, if anything, ordered and orderly. They say she "revealed all" to the *Daily Mail* (July 6, 2011), a British tabloid. Revealed all? Hmmm. Aren't some things better left to the imagination?

She believes that fat is beautiful. Debatable. And that it is healthy. Unlikely.

Although, face it, if she were trapped on a mountain ledge with no buffet around, she could live off herself for a century or 12.

The thing is, she's figured out food. This story has legs. Like it or not.

At least for now, the government of concern—if indeed there is one—figures it has bigger fish to fry than this New Jersey whale wannabe. Hard to believe, given the Western world's growing affection for the nanny state. So should the nanny state nag her fanny state?

All we can say is—with gritty guts and gargantuan gut, Donna does devour grub. And her time's not up! There is no finale on this overture to obesity, no last point in this longing for largeness, no ending in this exaltation of enormity, for conclusions are inconsequential, delusions—as compared to the porcine scene to be seen.

And hey, as for you naysayers? Lighten up.

Oops. Might have to scratch all this above. The home page of her official domain, donnasimpson.com, has a letter from her. She wants to backtrack. And slim down. She's had enough. Under "The Whole Truth" (February 22, 2012), she says, yes she did appear on the Tyra Banks show and yes, she admitted to wanting to gain weight, but that the hard numbers being bandied about were just so much media mumbo-jumbo.

Oh.

Chapter 62
In India, youth cigarette smoking causes a bidi cancer!

And everywhere...

Living off the land is a killer. In India young villagers are dying on the vine and twine—what with their surfeit of cigarette smoking.

It seems ignorance is *not* bliss and relying on homespun wisdom to set life right *is* the wrong move for health. So when someone says they are going to retreat back to nature tell-and-tweet them to shut up and stay put in the smog-filled city, where it's safer.

Says who?

Says Professor Prabhat Jha at the Centre for Global Health Research at St. Michael's Hospital in Toronto. One of his papers says that tobacco is the culprit for 40% of cancers in men and 20% in women. Should we in the West care and wring our hands at what the East is doing to itself?

Given that all the Western computer IT and programming jobs have stampeded to India, probably not. But the Western and Eastern scientific mind (except for the eco-freak climate warming geeks) craves reasoned thought and action leading to inexorable improved outcomes in health, mind, and spirit.

Having a country's health indices move backward just won't do.

But it will if nothing changes. The young are naturally rebellious, no matter the caste, class, culture, or country—and if they hear something is bad for them—well that's fodder for the fool.

India has lotsa smoking laws and admonishments. All are ignored when and where possible. That may piss off bureaucrats but it turns on the death industry: In 2010 an estimated one million folks were slated to be slain from smoking.

And the *New England Journal of Medicine*'s 900 snoops (non-medical field workers) who went to get the tobacco use scoop in India found that the men who smoked would stand a 20% greater chance of dying between the ages of 30 and 69 than would their non-smoking counterparts.

Indian men who inhale will never become old biddies because of, well, bidis.

What?

What the heck are bidis? Bidis are cigarettes produced by the Azadbidi Company, to the tune of 12 billion per year, for inhaling in India and beyond. They are exported to more than 122 countries.

Why do people in India—and everywhere else—like smoking bidis or other brands? (Azadbidi blows blatant marketing smoke rings, boasting the bidi blends perfection, taste, and quality.) The tendu leaf—instead of rolling paper—wraps up the bidi (or biri or beedi) and its tobacco, and is tightened with a string.

The bidi is saving the environment from the ruthless paper industry! And the tendu leaf has herbal properties. And—as a product of Indian industry—it had Gandhi's support.

Yet even the most adamant smoker admits it's a filthy habit. All but the obtuse or willfully blind know it's bad for your skin, lungs, heart, and self-esteem. Yet in India—where young people get cancer even sooner than in China, a remarkably rancid feat—they persist in inhaling death like there's no tomorrow.

People, despite the evident health hazards, get an inner personal psychological satisfaction from lighting up. Smoking also curbs appetites and that's a plus for those who want to look healthy without bothering to exercise. Sure they are flabby underneath, but clothes artfully draped will show them as svelte, not soft.

And to take a smoke break from work not only offers a fleeting release from tension but allows for feisty self-expression hinting of rebellion: Look at me. I'm a rebel, living on the edge, skirting society's authority. We think we look hot—or at least not as klutzy and clunky as we usually do.

The government of India, like most governments, fusses about health but suffers from bureaucratic overlap in minding its citizens. But one concerned official Indian department gets an A for a name that is so long winded you'll have to catch your breath after reading it. Hope you're not a smoker:

Department of Ayurveda, Yoga & Naturopathy, Unani, Siddha and Homeopathy (AYUSH).

Got that? Then get this: Smoke one to seven bidis per day and watch your mortality rate climb 25%. (Presumably, if you don't smoke an itty-bitty bidi, which contains about 1/4 the tobacco of a full-sized cigarette, in which case you'll stand a 25% lower chance of dying.)

Does Bollywood affect smoking? Do stilts make you taller? You bet Bollywood, a huge movie industry whose actors smoke, imprints bad habits on the young. It got so bad that the government tried to ban smoking in the movies. But the Delhi High Court turned that aside in 2009, saying it was censorious and a contravention of free speech.

Indian programmers have basically taken over the computer world. Newfound affluence, and a rapidly growing middle class, mean more money for cigarettes. Or maybe Indian IT experts chain smoke to relieve the pain of trying to teach stupid Westerners how to boot up their computers…

According to the study, more than 50% of smokers in India are illiterate. Nevertheless, a good chunk of smokers there *are* literate, and yet they are fueling their early demise.

The government is torn between protecting the health of citizens and protecting their own political necks: Tobacco growers vote and aid the economy. Discouraging them from either activity is not conducive to a long, healthy political life.

In the end, to save lives, India may need a personal, pleading, near-deathbed appeal to *stub out and smarten up*—perhaps from an Indian version of Hollywood star Yul Brynner (1920–1985), who made just such an anti-smoking commercial before his death. Then the impressionable may think twice before continuing or starting this vice. Failing that, Indian smoking statistics will continue to rise—as will avoidable, untimely deaths.

Chapter 63
China bans smoking

The laws in China and various other countries may have changed since this article was written. But the trend is clear: Everywhere, smoking is becoming more of a social stain and stigma. Governments are restricting, via legislation and admonition, its place in public spaces.

By reducing smoking, China is helping to curb its notorious pollution problems. It is cutting back on hydrogen cyanide, benzene, formaldehyde, acetone and even carbon monoxide, all of which are found in cigarettes. But what gives? China bans smoking? Is this wise? It has to be a lot wiser, and way nicer, than its *One Child* policy. If the left hand wants to curb population growth by restricting family member counts and the right hand decides more people should live via a curtailment of cigarettes, aren't the two diktats running at cross purposes?

Anyway, China has banned smoking in public places. Although punishments don't come hand in hand with illegally lighting up, it's only a matter of time. Now fellow citizens will be spared the mug-ugly lousy teeth and sallow skin of their fellow comrades. Looks good on them.

Lao Tzu, considered the founder of Taoism, said: "To know one's ignorance is the best part of knowledge." Smokers are smart enough to know they are stupid.

But what of governments? Do they think their scare tactic photos of lesions, boils, and gory gums on cigarette packages deter smokers and wannabees?

Yes, if we are to believe marketing researchers at the University of Arkansas, Villanova University, and Marquette University. Of course, they only surveyed approximately 500 smokers in the USA and in Canada. Could be, they were the only ones who could complete the survey without coughing up a lung.

The trend towards elimination of smoking is omnipresent. California used to lead the world in inventions but now, alas, leads only in interventions. But some laws, to prevent a person from persuading his progeny to smoke by preventing him from indulging in that habit, are probably a good thing. In stigmatizing and shunning smokers, the left-west coast of California may be onto something.

But if you don't want to catch this wave, and do want to light up, best go to Russia, setting your time machine to reverse. Before February 2013, more than four out of ten Russians were deemed smokers but now Vladimir Putin is putting on the brakes. As of June 2013, smoking will be banned on beaches, in playgrounds, and around entrances to workplaces, airports, stations, and ports. But diners will be able to wine and wheeze without whining, as cigarettes won't be banned in restaurants, on really long train trips, and in front of housing complexes until the next year.

The United States, for its part, has no Putin-style federal ban; smoking is legislated state-by-state, and the details of laws are broad and sometimes peculiar. Brazil's biggies, São Paulo and Rio, effective August 2009, banned smoking in all public places. Similarly, Canada has nixed nicotine in most indoor public places.

Heck, in Canada's most populous province, Ontario, you can't even smoke in your own car. Not if a kid younger than 16 is present. While smoking is socially snubbed, steep prices per pack, owing to outrageous federal and provincial taxation, have sent smuggling soaring. And roaring. At night. In very fast boats.

Like on the Akwesasne Indian reserve which straddles Ontario, Quebec, and New York State. Taxpayers and law enforcement agencies can point fingers all they want, but some estimate that nearly 50% of all cigarettes smoked in Canada come from illegal sources.

Why do people smoke? Why do people do half the crazy things they do to harm themselves? We haven't a clue. Test on Thursday. Still, smoking is legal in many places and tobacco farmers in southern Ontario, for example, are feeling the pinch, and are feeling they have been hung out to dry by overzealous governments.

But ultimate success to move these long time tobacco growers to different crops will take root as soon as the poppy is eradicated in Afghanistan as a cash crop.

If cigarettes are eradicated—would that eliminate the ardent, holier-than-thou, anti-smoking activists? Priggish, prudish, rude, and crude, they rank second on the slug-smug scale, just behind the anti-fur brigade. Lighten up and light up. A person, it used to be, had the inalienable right to wreck their life, and get "lit" every once in a while, if only to vex these patrolling pests. Just joshing. Perhaps.

Back to China. What caused the government's about-face against a national pastime for decades? The Olympics. Visitors might find the cultural norm of nearly 25% of Chinese hacking and spitting away unseemly. The new public ban on smoking came into force in Beijing in 2008.

But communist bravado and firepower only go so far. They tried to get the restaurants and bars to go along with this idea, and the latter promptly bucked it, so the government just trashed it. Tanks work better against students than against smokers and barkeeps. It's hard to change a culture where men would smoke even on jam-packed elevators. And the Chinese State Tobacco Monopoly Administration promotes tobacco like there's no tomorrow. And it keys in on men. While over 50% (other research offers a percentage nearer to 75%) of men partake in China, only about 4% of women do. Quite a discrepancy, due in part no doubt to boys being boys, meaning to be men…

And while no one knows what to expect from teens—other than that they will, figuratively and literally, roll their eyes at nearly everything a parent thinks, feels, speaks, and lives for—they do in fact watch, and yes, sometimes listen, to positive messages about the negative impact cigarettes have.

Because, there are *4,000* known chemical compounds (boy, it would be cool to see them listed, huh?) that are released when cigarettes are smoked. Speaking of cancer, 69 of the 4,000 chemicals are reckoned to cause cancer.

If you quit smoking, you lift your life. If you don't, you lose it, and that goes double for the 2,000 Chinese who are dying like weeds daily, from the effects of smoking.

Chapter 64
The UN's Olivier de Schutter declares obesity a systemic epidemic

The United Nations has no problem with keeping Syria on a human rights committee, but it does have a big problem with what you are eating. This just shows what a complete joke that fetid organization is, and why nobody with half a brain should take whatever it says even half seriously.

It's hard to say which is dumber and more insulting, UNESCO's basic whitewashing of Syria's slaughter against its own folks, or the UN's special reporter on the right to food, Olivier de Schutter, getting down and dirty, hectoring us Neanderthals the world over, for not living up to the UN's platter standards.

With Syria, UN unobtrusiveness in action is front and center. With food and you, UN intrusiveness is right in your face. It's a disgrace.

So what specifically is the story on this new food cop? On March 6th, 2012, Mr. de Schutter presented his food factoids to the 19th session of the UN Human Rights Council (the report was published August 4th, 2011). Terribly earnest and perhaps well meaning, his arguments would have been far more germane to the "Right to Food" and human rights in general if he had talked down on why Bashar al-Assad should not be figuratively barbequing the Syrian citizenry.

Oops, sorry. De Schutter is the *Special Rapporteur* on the *Right to Food*. The French gives it a nice twist, no? It oozes in self-importance and bursts with pomposity. Frustratingly, if this sentence from his report is any indication, he can't write. Can anyone explain what's being said?

"This report identifies the issues raised by the expansion of contract farming and notes seven areas in which Governments and firms could ensure that it results in pro-poor outcomes and contributes to the full realization of the right to food."

Does it make sense for seven areas to result in pro-poor outcomes at once, yet contribute to the full realization of the right to food? Does he get bulimic reading his own drivel?

De Schutter, according to some, is unabashedly systemic: he wants to politicize food and have the UN look after your meals with the same care, competence, and class it has looked after enhancing and enabling world peace since WWII's end in 1945.

In 2012, for those eco-freak North Americans who like their luminaries world-weary dreary, you could have caught de Schutter snooping in Canada from May 5th to May 15th, lecturing Canadians on food. Canadians are getting fatter by the nano-second. Food is not a problem. Food is already "a right" there: they're right into the food. But de Schutter doesn't appreciate Canadians', or the world's, choices in food. They offend his sensibilities.

Shoulda been a French waiter.

Basically, because the USA is the UN's biggest donor—at about 22% of the budget (though it's not always on time with its dues) and because the USA, despite its massive debt problems and foreign adventure escapades, is still the most admired, successful, country going—and because this is a UN representative, don't forget, the obesity epidemic is declared to be America's fault.

Or at least the fault of American private industries making and marketing food. Olivier de Schutter, his resume replete with governmental and NGO affiliation accomplishments, may be a smarty. He's most assuredly a snarky, figuring us fat heads are either too weak or too dumb to fend off food companies with their mes-sages of eat this, and now eat this—in triplicate!

De Schutter doesn't fault the citizen for lack of self-discipline. He finds no solace in an individual exercising his free will to decide what is crammed down the old chute. The right to pick—unencumbered by governmental fiat—just won't do, and wouldn't be tolerated if he gets his way.

He wants the basically bankrupt American government to launch a spending spree on an advertising avalanche, telling people to eat... local fresh food. The right to food, it appears, is not a true, unqualified right to food—but only a tightly approved right to food, ordained by de Schutter himself.

"Nutritional failures are political." Those wrong-headed words are his. In reality, nutritional failures are largely personal, except for when a United Nations member country is intentionally starving a portion of its population. Then, okay, it's politi-cal—but given the refusal of the United Nations, thanks to China and Russia, to protect the oppressed and the offed in Syria—it sure isn't going to send the cavalry in if some despicable dictator decides his country's people, deemed wretched and wasteworthy, should waste away.

His treatise isn't a call to resolve food foul-ups, it's a blatant power grab. Both obesity and starvation are blamed on the global food system, whatever that means, and on political inertia. Cuba, under Fidel Castro's rotten reign, has had lots of political "ertia" and lotsa lousy harvests.

The old USSR, the Soviet Union, with the might of the Kremlin command economy under Joseph Stalin and his successors, couldn't even feed its own people, despite having the Ukrainian breadbasket as a vast source of food. It did, however, intentionally starve millions of Ukrainians in a genocide known as the Holodomor.

No matter. De Schutter has learned nothing from history or from the events of today. He still looks for solutions from government bureaucracy.

He's sorta right on one point. Children *are* amenable and susceptible to the blandishments of junk food advertising. But this is where parents step in. He seems to view most children as being on their own, without any defenders or intermediaries who step in to distract them from hard-sell product pitches. And if the kids were truly on their own, they wouldn't have the bucks to buy chips and candy anyway.

He blathers that we live in an "*obesogenic environment.*" Not sure what that means, but it sounds scary enough to make impressionable, susceptible adults succumb to his wants. He avers that it's "too easy to choose bad calories." But is *big government* micro-management of food likely to lead to a healthy diet, including vitamin-rich but perishable foods?

Perish the thought.

Chapter 65
Disney's "Habit Heroes" are a big anti-obesity zero

Fat jokes should not be for kids

Has Disney hit rock bottom with *Lead Bottom*? Lead Bottom is a gold blob with a bloated gargantuan gut, huger than a sumo wrestler on a burger binge, and a face as unattractive as all get out. If you ask Disney, Lead Bottom and his villainous counterparts in fat crime—including the sultry *Sweet Tooth*, *The Snacker* (a plump maiden who looks like a wisecracker), *Control Freak* (a menacing dark black robotic monster), *Ice Cappuccino* (a cool looking dude), and the slovenly, *Insecura*—are all bad-habit characters who must be crushed by heroes like *Callie Stenics* and *Will Power.*

Disney has joined the war against obesity, and these characters, presented in an anti-obesity exhibit, offer messages zestier than any dry-as-"dry toast, please" from the health and nutrition crowd. They have the potential, if not to wake up wide kids to their plight, at least to put a burr under the saddle of the anti-obesity orators who are currently riding high, and render them aghast. The orators are not amused.

In fact, they're confused and incensed, pissed even, that Disney would use such graphic displays to, in their opinion, shame and blame—and essentially name—obese youngsters as folks worthy of derision.

But do the kids really see it that way? Overprotective worrywarts fear that shame will cause tykes with tender psyches, and still-developing emotional coping strategies, to retract and withdraw. And, who knows, maybe they will balloon even more—newly rankled with misery and chagrin.

Or shaming could very well work. It could jolt the obese into taking matters into their own hands. To taking the steps necessary to change habits and do whatever else is needed to fly right and get slight.

Take The Glutton, for example. This thoroughly gross tub of lard, in a pinstripe suit tight enough to burst, with a mug only a venal fat-cat banker would love, might be the catalyst for a child to say: If I keep this up—I'm going to *be* that portly pig someday.

One could argue that the images are not so much to shame as to scare. And getting scared straight, or slim, could help kids arrest a near-criminal rise in obesity, among themselves at least, and perhaps their parents.

Disney has an audience bigger than any professor of picky-picayune food management from Rodomontade University. And if Disney didn't, pun intended, use larger-than-life personas to get their message out, Disney wouldn't be Disney. They'd be just another boring, run of the mill, ho-hum, dum-de-dum public service announcement that would get zapped faster than a pop tart in a nuclear reactor.

The creatures above, and others like *Drama Queen*, who gossips way too much for Disney's Habit Heroes, are *supposed to be* shot down by the kids. Killing off the bad guys, bad apples, sounds like a lot of fun—and kids can quite easily separate reality from fantasy. So they will know enough *not* to jeer at a chubby friend coming up the walk.

But Disney apparently got out of the kitchen, for it couldn't stand the heat, fueled by withering criticism from the likes of the Binge Eating Disorder Association, the National Association of Anorexia Nervosa and Associated Disorders, and Dr. Yoni Freedhoff, an assistant professor of family medicine.

Didn't somebody say that any publicity is good publicity? Why should Disney cower in the wake of censure from an assistant professor? Has Disney no backbone, no balls? Disney has closed the exhibit "for the time being." It closed faster than a bigot's mind in 2011 (but reopened later, tentatively, in 2012).

One wonders if Disney's Habit Heroes, who occupy the virtual world of the Disney Web site and are on the smart phone as a Habit Heroes mobile, will none-theless meet an ignoble premature death.

Catch your breath. Freedhoff thinks that the Disney Habit Heroes stereotype obesity. Stereotyping and stigmatization are two of the more unpleasant actions we humans do, but they won't kill someone as quickly as obesity will—as many medical practitioners can testify.

Look, whatever society has tried up to now, in the West and in the Third World, hasn't worked a tinker's damn in stemming or slowing the rise of fatties among us. Time to overturn the apple cart of accepted nostrums and try some new, albeit lurid, tactics to make the most impressionable among us take a good, hard look at themselves.

Has the past few years of nanny parenting and endless praise of our progeny worked? Has showering kids with computers and TVs in their rooms helped? Kids feel more entitled than ever before—and one of their first entitlements is appar-ently to forego self-examination and refuse to listen to urgent health messages from anyone else.

Freedhoff may have a point when he says (paraphrasing here) that the last thing a tot wants to see while whirling, twirling, and touring at the Epcot theme park, is a reminder of the body they already view as horrible or at least as a target of criticism or teasing.

Are Disney's Habit Heroes such a big zero in the fight against obesity? Surely their shock value might turn some kids' lives around…

No child or adult should mosey through life with rose-colored glasses on, searching for nirvana, a bliss with all in perfect place, and nothing negative or amiss. Life is full of ugly truths. An honest reality check of our personal challenges is the height of responsibility. It arms a person for the good fight against, in this case, fat. Yes, depression about a situation can, in extreme cases, lead to suicide. The thing is, depression about a problem only leads to suicide in people who are already inclined to suicidal depression. If children show any such signs, they should be treated promptly. But one can't make public policy for whole nations based on rare, acute problems. And yes, having one's self-image punctured by Disney's cartoonish oafs and boorish miscreants is a bummer. But self-awareness—even if it hurts—might be a necessary basic step to identifying a problem, then setting out to do something about it.

Chapter 66
Parent or child obesity as a weapon in family court wars

Well it had to happen sooner or later. The courts are now hosting parent-child obesity wars. Horrors.

Parenting, we know is a pretty tough job; there is no learner's manual and no graduated licensing system; one minute you are footloose and fancy-free, and the next minute you are buried under six kids because you gobbled up super duper fertility pills, thinking they were candy.

With parenting comes relationships, and they can be harsh even when running smoothly. They are brutal when sputtering badly, leaving togetherness a smoldering wreck. Fortunately, the courts will hear, and they are near.

Now how do the chubby fit in? Well, child obesity is now being factored into custody judgments and child welfare decisions. Calculation by caliper and custody conclusions by court is with us. If you overfeed your kid, according to their pinch-an-inch gut instincts—you just might see your ex get custody.

Don't believe me? In 2008, an Ontario family court cited obesity as a reason for removing a child from the parental home, after it determined that the mother was contributing to the child's weight gain and was oblivious to the necessary medical regime (*National Post*, March 4, 2008).

Medical regime? Sounds a tad dictatorial, no? How was mom contributing to her child's weight gain? Was she doing crazy stuff, like feeding the child again and again?

Well we can't be sure because there is a publication ban on the case. But another case, which offers more freedom for the press, certainly points to where things are headed: A *nine-year* custody battle, again in Ontario, centered on the ability of each respective parent to best feed twins who were classified as obese. So maybe drastic action was required.

Both parents in the prolonged custody battle considered themselves key to their kids' health. These children had been in "intensive hospital-based obesity programs" most of their lives (*National Post*, March 4, 2008).

A childhood obesity expert, Dr. Glenn Berall, Chief of Pediatrics at the North York General Hospital, swung for the fences, opining that the court should choose the parent who "had demonstrated the ability to comply with a prescribed weight-management program and *to restrict access to the parent who did not reasonably comply.*"

For those keeping score, the mom won. And this was despite the fact that the kids gained excess weight while with their mom. Dr. Berall testified that the brother and sister lost weight while with their dad. In this case, obesity—clearly—wasn't the deciding factor in awarding the mother primary custody.

But is Dr. Berall serious about his injunction to *restrict access to the parent who did not reasonably comply*? That's pretty severe. Is this where we, as a society, want to be led? What's next—unwanted, unsolicited, unnecessary raids by anti-obesity storm troopers arriving in the dead of the night to check for offending items in fridges, cupboards, and waste bins?

Those who argue that society has a duty to intervene and cart children away from home when they are severely obese, point out that if the kids were starving, most of us would have no qualms about rescuing them. For sure, however, under-nourished and overnourished, as reference points, are subjective and vary from culture to culture. It's a can of worms, in other words. Why, for example, should a foster home be deemed better for the obese child? Is the foster parent supposed to be especially gifted in these matters? If the child is older, there is a good chance that he or she can and will simply resist any slimming program, if so motivated. So what is gained by taking the child out of a familiar environment?

In another twist, an Ottawa, Ontario, man who weighed 380 pounds (as of 2012) was denied access to his two boys by the Royal Ottawa Hospital's family court clinic (*CBC News,* June 19, 2012). He says he's mobile, and he's proven his determination to lose weight already, losing about 180 pounds. He loves his kids. And he was peeved. He hadn't seen his kids (around five and six years old) since 2011.

The hospital seems to get its marching orders from the Child and Family Services Act. Reader comments on the story/scandal brought up other factors that may underlie denial of access. The man was an admitted previous marijuana user who has also refused gastric bypass surgery because he wants to lose weight through his own willpower and methods. Where are the kids now? They are with the Children's Aid Society. Where's mom? Well apparently, the ex-wife had the kids but they were seized when she was hospitalized with a suspected drug overdose.

It seems that those that want to snatch kids away from obese parents view obesity as a moral failing, a scourge. But what if genetic history or medication have an impact on a court participant's body size? And does being fat clearly render a parent unable or unwilling to show and demonstrate parental supervision and love? (This assumes the parent is not bedridden, too big to move.) Fortunately (or not, depending on your point of view), in the previously mentioned nine-year custody battle, obesity wasn't the determining factor.

But if the trend leans to smearing obese parents as, no pun intended, unfit parents, what do we do with the little ones whose parents smoke cigarettes?

Puff on this not-too-risky prediction: With opinions all over the board as to whether courts should separate children from parents if the child or the parent is obese, cases will only multiply, given that obesity rates for both children and adults are shooting up pretty well everywhere.

Chapter 67
Two hundred-pound Ohio boy taken from mother

How would you like it if your kid was on the honor roll, but was yanked away from you, the mother, because said kid weighs 200 pounds? And now you get visitation hours with him—a measly two hours per week?

That appears to be the plight of a Cleveland, Ohio, mother whose son is now in government care. Boy, oh boy, that doesn't sound good. Look at how the federal and state governments have let debts balloon with no similar level of concern for the children who will have to pay them off. But this is a local jurisdiction so...

So get this, the government was thinking of finding a foster home with a fitness trainer. Why don't they just give funds to the mom with the proviso that they be spent on such?

No one will deny that the 200-pound (90.71 kg) Ohio boy is *way too big for his age*. He's only eight years old. Government charts say he should weigh around 60 pounds (27.21 kg). But with child obesity rates soaring throughout the USA (and in Ohio, 12% of third graders are deemed severely obese), do the powers that be really want to start a rotund-child relocation program? Won't it weigh (no pun intended) emotionally on mother and son?

The mother is not a basket case. Okay, right now she's bonkers with grief, but she loves her son, as most mothers do. She has tried to get him to eat less and exercise more. She works with her child and works as a substitute elementary school teacher too. It's not like she's a druggie or something.

Government standards for every facet of human activity change faster than a politician's convictions, when tested. Today, 200 pounds merits the heave-ho in Cleveland. But what if next year, by fiat, the bureaucrat of fat declares that 190 pounds should be enough to do the trick, and trigger the obesity police to drag (or lift, slowly) the offending child away?

Not only do governments and public administrations continually tinker with rules and regulations, they often work at cross-purposes with each other. In Ontario, Canada, there are fat kids. Yet at the Earl Beatty elementary school, they banned soccer balls, volleyballs, and basketballs from the playground. How does that help kids work off that excess energy and weight?

It doesn't. Safety 1, Kid's fun 0, Kid's obesity 10.

So kids, being smart and adaptable, belly up to the TV or PC.

Right now fat is no fad, it's "out." But what happens when Tonga invades—will the portly be put on pedestals? All this government calculation, machination, and deliberation to remake this 200-pound Grade Three boy into a new approved boy-toy reminds one of darker times, when Joe Stalin was remaking Russians into the "new Soviet man."

What happens if the kid flunks at losing weight? Do they drown him in the river with a bag of kittens? What is the last stop after parental and nanny-state solutions fail?

Governments are more concerned about a person's perfectly legal snacking habits then they are with the sacking habits of G-20 and Occupy Wall Street protestors. The OWS kids were hailed. If you are a tubby tyke, you're nailed—ripped from the bosom of the family, all on account of cupcakes. Them's the breaks...

So our pudgy protagonist is in foster care—no doubt with caregivers who will devote all requisite attention, and shower the boy with love, as would his family.

Not.

County social workers just didn't like his weight. No debate.

Well actually there was lots of debate—for 20 months, says agency administrator Patricia Rideout, before the expulsion was ordained under the proviso of "medical neglect." If mom was a doctor, this might be a fine basket to put governmental legal wares in, but she's just a mother. And currently, her lawyer says, the boy's not in any imminently life-threatening situation. Put another way—being alive—his chances of dying are as good as yours or mine.

Even Juvenile Public Defender Sam Amata is taken aback at this state-sanctioned *kid*nap. "But what risk became imminent? When did it become an immediate problem?" (*Cleveland Plain Dealer*, November 26, 2011).

Apparently Cuyahoga County doesn't have set guidelines for the removal of kids. It draws straws and this kid drew the short one. Just kidding. Mary Louise Madigan of the Department of Children and Family Services says the "medical neglect" label seemed to fit.

According to Cuyahoga County's official Web site (as of mid-2013), if they decide the parents aren't up to snuff, they'll sniff around to see if relatives have that indefinable royal jelly. If the relatives don't make the grade, which we have to assume happened here, a foster home is the next best choice. But—as the site adds—these are temporary arrangements.

How can mom get her child back? "Ohio law requires that DCFS file a case plan with Juvenile Court prior to the adjudicatory hearing (trial), but no later than 30 days after the complaint was filed or the child was placed in care. The case plan outlines requirements the parents must fulfill in order to regain custody of their child."

And what requirements would those be? Might they be a general pledge to double down on one's efforts and give that old 110% to help reduce the kid's weight, or might she have to submit a dietary plan—that meets the approval of the social workers? Will she have to slap an electronic bracelet onto the boy so the social workers can be alerted if the young fellow so much as enters a 50-yard radius of any public establishment that contains a scintilla of junk foods—in bulk or in trace amounts—in which case a SWAT team can scoot the unsuspecting youngster away from possible, potential, self-administered abuse and neglect?

For *abuse* and *neglect* are key words to this hand-wringing, overwrought, caring crowd. Starving a child—that's abuse. But now, seemingly, raising an obese child is deemed abhorrent by a rapidly fattening society—and that's abuse too.

Great Britain has also caught the kid's-too-big bug: five youngsters were taken from their families in 2013 for being deemed too portly.

Chapter 68
Teenage waist land - belly band surgery

Today's teenagers, like teenagers of eras past, are on the cutting edge of trends. Except now they are taking this cutting edge stuff literally. Forget the hula hoop, the twist, body piercing and tattoos. The kids of today are careening out of control and are driving their chassis into the obesity shop where they can get their extra bumpers and fenders hacked, sawed, and otherwise cut off.

Hospitals in the USA are licking their chops over the profit potential from this surge in elective surgery. From *New York Daily News* (December 4, 2006), we learned:

A top New York hospital has become one of the first in the nation to open a center specifically to perform drastic "belly band" surgery on overweight kids. The Center for Adolescent Bariatric Surgery at Morgan Stanley Children's Hospital of New York-Presbyterian has already performed six operations on teens. Four more will have it by year's end and about 40 kids—now in a six-month weight loss program—may be eligible by spring. More than 30% of America's teens are overweight. 15% teens are obese, according to the American Obesity Association.

(And this is just one more darned thing for harried parents to worry about.)

Should parents and their progeny be eagerly salivating to sign on the dotted line for such drastic surgical acts? This remedy may reduce youth obesity stats but experts might recommend simpler, less invasive, solutions like: Take a hike.

Literally.

Hit the road. Parents should put a deep freeze on kids' computer and TV time, and figure out athletic alternatives. But until these and other options are advocated and introduced, here is how things are playing out in hospitals, again from the *New York Daily News:*

"We've come around to the opinion that it's actually much better to try and intervene very early," said center director Dr. Jeffrey Zitsman.

Another hospital—New York University Medical Center—has already performed nearly 90 gastric banding procedures. A handful of hospitals perform the surgery on adolescents, but Morgan Stanley, NYU Medical Center and the

University of Illinois at Chicago are the only hospitals approved by the Food and Drug Administration to operate on children as young as 14, Zitsman said.

One doctor described the surgery, in which a silicone band around the top of the stomach creates a pouch that holds only a small amount of food (so that the patient feels full and stops eating) as "a radical step" and not an everyday solution for oversize teens. Other doctors have been more critical, including Julio Teixeira, chief of minimally invasive surgery at St. Luke's Hospital:

With procedures costing $15,000 to $30,000, "bariatric surgery is an oil gusher for hospitals… The interest is going to be there for developing a pediatric program," Teixeira said.

Some doctors reluctantly support surgery in order to avoid or reduce related medical problems like diabetes and sleep apnea, as well as psychologically damaging social stigma.

"I tell everyone right upfront that we're not interested in selling operations. This is a program. The surgery is just one piece of it," Zitsman said. "If society would put us out of business, we'd be happy to close."

If you say so, Dr. Zitsman. But any way you look at it, this is a new and, ahem, growing frontier where how far and wide it can go are limited only by girths. There *has* to be a better way. While walking, for example, is not trendy or chic, it is tried and true, and is still a cure that costs little and pays off big.

Chapter 69

Giuliano Stroe is The World's Strongest Boy (Guinness World Records Says So)

Giuliano Stroe is a far cry indeed from the kids whose obesity problems have made it to the courts. I include his profile just to show the variety that can be found in human life on this planet, and as something of a demonstration, perhaps, that things *can* be different. This kid hand walks for the pleasure of millions. He amazes us with air push ups. Giuliano was a tiny, mighty tyke of seven years old in July 2011, when I first wrote about him:

He plays and works—and excels with—weights in the family's gym in Ciuresti, Romania. He's ripped. He's cute. The camera loves him, and so does YouTube: Stroe's videos have been viewed countless times.

Now countless times and one.

With his winning wink for the camera, he's a natural born bit of a ham, but it's refreshing to see a *ham-who-can*. So yes, we should we give a big hand to Giuliano's handstand pushups. *From a high bar.*

Which brings us to *your* darling child. Is your kid a mighty mouse or a meek squeak?

But before you dash out and buy barbells and that high bar nobody's been begging for, and install Stroe's gymnasium, replete with chalk and mats, with you yourself acting as the spotter—should you take a deep breath and ponder?

Is resistance training safe for kids? A CrossFit gym in Calgary, Alberta, thinks so, and they're not the only ones. Many fitness clubs have shifted resources to youngsters. *Bloomberg BusinessWeek* tells us (July 14, 2011).

Over the past five years pre-adolescent and teen memberships have increased by 2.9 percent annually—and the 6-to-11 age category has almost doubled since 2005.

But what of the risk with pre-pubescent children hoisting iron, causing premature bone fusion (epiphyseal fusion), ending in irreversibly stunted growth? The devil is in the details. Could a kid's body, hormonally and structurally, handle high intensity push-to-failure routines?

No.

But age appropriate weights, as defined by a certified trainer, and a gradual increase in weight amounts or repetition, say on a weekly basis, may be safe.

Time for the ominous, obligatory warning: Consult a doctor or a physician. Don't even think or plan anything at all in life before chatting with your medical practitioner. To keep kids safe from all hurts, hangnails, and hang-ups, don't have those kids. If you must have kids, make sure they are plastic wrapped in a sealant protector with body armor worn at all times.

But hey, seriously, if you want to leap, sing, and dance, and you are aged 2.5 to 5, a gym like CrossFit may be for you. Plead with your parents. With the jumping around comes a great workout for those legs and, later possibly, weights may be added in. The singing and dancing is for the reality competition down the road...

Back on track. Foolishness sidelines little ones. Bending the rules of common sense leaves injured kids on the outside looking in... Remember Giuliano Stroe is one in a billion.

Enter golf's numero Uno Jack Nicklaus and pitching star John Smoltz. They're working with doctors and other great athletes in the just-launched Stop Sports Injuries campaign to warn about the ways in which overexertion can lead to injury. Could mighty Giuliano have fallen prey to such calamity?

He might have, if he and his dad didn't practice a "balance is best" philosophy. Beaming in on one favorite sport, playing the be-jesus out of it all year round, ends with one bummer of a burnout. Mentally, you end up hating the sport and physically, you're looking at overuse injury because muscles are not allowed to rest and recuperate from the rigors of a season spent in the same old action-and-reaction.

Dad, now assisted by the ubiquitous social media, keeps an eye on Giuliano. He's *okay*. Another plus? Giuliano mixes in gymnastics with weights, albeit from the age of two. Phew.

And weight training is not listed as an injurious sport for kids. That could be because so few kids do it to the exclusion of all else.

But for kids going steady with: baseball, basketball, cheerleading, dancing, football, gymnastics, running, soccer, softball, swimming, tennis, and volleyball—well obviously blend your pastimes, no matter what the type—and for heaven's sake—take a break.

So even while Giuliano breaks the world record for "Air Push Ups" his father, Iulian, has both feet on the ground. He supervises each session. Moreover, when Giuliano wants to kick back and goof around, that's encouraged, and it's A-OK.

Fortunately too, gymnastics has nearly everything: balance, strength, flexibility, coordination, and agility, lending to an all-round training of the body. And while starting at two years of age is incredible, many kids are in gymnastics by the time they hit the ripe old age of five.

What is it about Romania and gymnasts anyway? Remember Nadia Elena Comăneci? At the tender age of 14, she wowed the world and blew away the judges with a perfect routine in the uneven bars at the Montreal Olympics in 1976. It was the first perfect score given out in modern Olympic Gymnastics history.

Giuliano's a little young to make Olympic history but he is just fine for the Guinness Book of World Records. He's been notarized and immortalized for his "fastest ever ten metre (33 feet) hand-walk with a weight ball between his legs."

Giuliano Stroe, in life and limb, is a special case, an exceptional case. He's got the good genes with the great gumption. He has proper coaching with a pro-play attitude. He's been sprinkled with a dollop of luck and with other indefinables that make up such an A-One athlete. Read of him on Facebook. Gawk in awe, in shock at his strength, on YouTube. No matter the forum, the wunderkind is here to stay. And, lo and behold, something tells us his exertions and efforts are *by far* not yet over, the complete story told. For the kid's blessed—the kid's bold.

Chapter 70
2012 Calgary Stampede Bull Riding event—no BS!

So you think you're fit?

Would you have a cow at the very thought of riding a bull? Darn tootin' you would. You'd be nuts if you didn't, but cowboys who ride these 1,800 pound beasts are hard nuts to crack.

Does one, in a drug-addled daze or a coin tossing phase, choose bull riding over actuarial accounting? Does that make sense? And does one make decent dough, not-bad cents in this Western sport? Well, the World Finals of bull riding is the big daddy of greenbacks, with a total purse of $2 million plus, and as I write this, the Calgary Stampede 2012 is almost upon us...

Besides a cowboy's gut and grit, there are gobs of technical niceties needed to survive and thrive for 8 successfully seated seconds atop a bucking bull. The bull is 50% of the duo and of the total mark of 100. And if, in the judges' opinion, a bull lacked the requisite bucking bitchiness, the cowboy can get a "reride" on another bull.

Yet the cowboy's chances hang by a thread: a rope. There has to be some "give" in the rope, allowing the rider atop even the rankest of bulls to get "out in front." When there is not enough "give" in the rope to allow the hand to turn over, the cowboy is effectively handcuffed, as opposed to being ripe for a straitjacket. World Champion bull rider, Hall-of-Famer Gary Leffew, talks of a "narrow block" which is a band of leather of lesser width, just beside the looped rope handle. It allows for greater maneuverability. Listen, when the bull is about to buck you to kingdom come, you don't want to get hung up.

So you gotta get a grip on this sport. Really. It's an underhanded operation, and your butt should be forward of the one "underhand" that has hold of the handle. The tail of the rope, gripped tightly, must still be loose enough to let the hand move forward, and roll up on the knuckles. That hand *must* be able to free itself from the grip by merely [?!] loosening, allowing the handle and the rope tail to be released from the palm. Leffew talks of the "House of Pain," a cowboy experiences when he rides behind the rope. Leffew swears by (and sells) the Hotman Bull Rope which helps that rider to get out in that out-in-front sweet spot.

Now what about that other, loose hand? If you wanna be a winner, and not get disqualified, your free hand is *not* free to touch either the bull or yourself.

And don't tie yourself down with lousy practice tactics either. According to Leffew, training on the mechanical Mighty Bucky/El Toro is exactly what you don't want to do, for the robotic action is not like the real live reaction of a bull.

Not surprisingly, any time you mess with a bull, there's going to be BS because get this: some bull owners think disreputable cads are spiking up bulls' suppers with anabolic steroids. Wouldn't this be like adding speedballs to a druggie's repertoire? Is this tweak really necessary?

No. The best "juicy" bucking bull style is based on Charlie Plummer's "Plummer" breed/mix of (often) a Brahma, Texas Longhorn, and English White Park. Add in the irritant of the flank straps (which don't touch the genitals) and, most important, top it all off with the mean temper of an individual bull. Reputable BBB's who make up the NBBA, that is, Bucking Bull Breeders who make up the National Bucking Bull Association, will reassure you of all this.

Got it? Now get on the bull. What's a good bull for you? Ideally, the perfect bull should be a bitter pill, with all the venom a typical mother-in-law can muster. The bull must want to buck and toss you off like Elizabeth Taylor cast off spouses. But don't lollygag about once you hit dirt. Skedaddle. Otherwise—unless the rodeo bull clowns are up to snuff—your stuff will be gored by the bull's horns and hind hooves.

Wanna wow the judges? Come to the bucking bash with bells on. Howzzat? Yes, two bells clanging underneath the bull accentuate the motion and commotion, and alert all that you are in the throes of a once-in-a-lifetime ride, and not yet thrown. A smaller bell banging against a bigger one works best. Just hope the judges aren't deaf. (But even if the whole grandstand is hard of hearing, everyone will see that you, the bull rider, are one crazy cat.)

And it's much better to have a braided bell handle rather than a brass ring. It is snug against the bull's brisket so the bull will be free of pain, allowing it to let loose on you with enough twists and torques to do Elvis Presley proud.

American Shane "Dr. Proctor" Procter—the 2008 Toughest Cowboy reality TV winner—sure did the 2011 Calgary Stampede proud, taking home the bacon as bull riding champion, earning $100,000 atop Canadian Finals Rodeo Champion bull, "Bomb's Away." But you gotta figure, if Bombs Away turned up at the pay counter, he'd get a bundle of cash too. (Douglas Duncan won the bull riding honors for the 2010 Calgary Stampede.)

As for the 2012 Calgary Stampede's bull riding event, the most dangerous, spiciest event on the menu, here's food for thought: Between bulls tougher-than-nails and cowboys who chew cement and spit out gravel, the whole Wildcard Saturday and Showdown Sunday shebang ought to appeal, gol dang, to every bull riding fan's palate.

And that's no bull.

And here's no bull either. Buckoff. That's what would have happened to you if you dared to try to ride the 1700 pound, mound of a bad-ass bull, Bushwacker. Bushwacker, consecutively, bucked the f- -k out of 42 of the bravest and toughest hombres bucked them nearly into outer space, as they tried to ride this beast for 8 seconds. Bushwacker is the 2013 World Champion Bull.

No bull. That's a bull.

Chapter 71
Pamplona—The running of the bulls

(This piece was written in 2011. Much below is tongue in cheek—which should in no way hide the fact that this is one dangerous event. In this year's 2013 running, one man was gored to death.)

The Running of the Bulls in Pamplona, Spain, is not fit for man or beast, which is why both do it. The bull does it because he is ordered to. The man does it because he is disordered.

The bull has an unusually bad day. First, the run, a weird stampede among strangers, sets the bull off in more ways than one. And second, once the strange sprint on skinny streets is done, the bull will be done too, courtesy of the matador, in that evening's bullfight.

And, to add ignominy to fatality, the bulls have to run the streets with oxen— eunuchs—the latter hired to keep the bulls on the straight and narrow, as it were.

Lots of prayer is involved. The bulls pray for a miracle hoping against hope they won't get pole-axed by the matador. (If they put up a grand fight that night, their prayers are answered and they are *indultado*, that is, pardoned.) Man prays because, face it, anyone who wears a white pant-shirt ensemble, sashayed by a red belt, fully aware that 15 souls have already been bull-voted off Spain through gruesome deaths, needs all the help he can get.

Pamplona itself sure doesn't need help. It is *the* premier showcase for this event, though there are towns in Spain and Mexico that ape the action. Also, Ireland has a running of wild boars, and no, we aren't talking politicians.

Speaking of politics, People for the Ethical Treatment of Animals (PETA) cares about animals like nobody's business—except that, when they do care about animals, it's everyone's business. They feel that, since they don't like the bull running, no silly billy should be allowed to pitter patter around in it. Too bad, so sad.

What's needed to run amok? Luck, a functioning body, a malfunctioning brain, an age over 18, and no booze on your breath. An ability to run like the dickens for 903 yards is also handy.

But don't wear your dandy Sunday best—and don't freak out when your whites turn red. Okay, flip out if the red is your blood. But chances are, and these are mighty good odds, you'll be showered in red, thanks to a soaking in Sangria. You might also be flaked with flour, marinated in mustard, and splattered with eggs just for good measure.

It's all part of the fun. Often the mayor and city council ahem, egg the participants on from a balcony above.

Viva! in Spanish and *Gora!* in Basque mean, roughly, let's get it on. It is mixed with a benediction to Saint Fermin. He's dead but his role of co-patron of Navarre and of this *encierro*, this race, is very much alive.

"Travel advisory" takes on a whole new meaning for those that choose to scamper ahead of quite irked bulls. The Running of the Bulls is bathed in ritual and washed in spirits (for those not running), and the whole thing is steeped in tradition (the tradition of total tempestuousness). But those that get out—entrails intact—will swear to all that this just isn't another run-of-the-mill day.

No kidding. It is probably the only time you would ever run going in two directions at once. Your feet and most of your body head forwards while your head heads backwards, craning to see how what you know full well is coming after you is coming along with that. It isn't easy to have brain and body utterly bisected, but maybe that helps; you pretty well have to be out of your mind to even *think* of doing this. Not everything goes according to plan. Bulls are farouche and finicky, and don't cotton to being herded along narrow, slippery cobblestone streets surrounded by screaming citizens and tourists (not to mention the wails of sirens) so they'll do 180s and turn—on *you*.

Keep a wide berth. Even though that's impossible in a sea of thrashing legs and a field of flailing arms.

It's festive, it's congestive—restive—and if you need a digestive after galloping over pools of blood (which does not deter shopkeepers from opening up right after the big splash bull-dash is done) you can settle your tummy and watch your lore on a big screen, thanks to instant replay. Yummy.

Later at the Plaza Castillo, groups that *actually came together to undertake this caper* will do a surreptitious head count. If you do a count and find you are a party of one, then you are probably in a hospital being interviewed, intravenous inconveniences and all, with your remembrances rolling out via YouTube.

Take this in. The end offers no respite—for bull or man. In fact there's a squeeze play to finish things off. "It is the downward sloping chute into the plaza, but the tunnel comes before the plaza and that is one scary place, as the sound echoes and it goes from 10 lanes to five, so the squeeze causes some pileups. One mozo was killed by suffocation, at the bottom of a pile." (*La Prensa,* June 6, 2008).

The Running of the Bulls is birthed in bulls bred for aggression, intelligence, strength, and stamina. It ends in their running, every July, with rapscallions bred for nothing much. It is not just a spectacle, but a snippet of how life should or should not be lived; not just a voyeur sport, but a voyage into the avoidable but un-voidable; not just a microcosm of the mysteriousness of life, but is a macrocosm of all that is positively mental about it.

'Nuff said. On with the show. Go, Bulls, go!

Chapter 72
Catania World Fencing Championships 2011. En garde!

Don't sit on the fence. Try this sport on for size. You'll get the point, right quick.

Will Italy lunge, parry, and riposte to first place in the World Fencing Championships 2011? They won in 2010, and this year's championship is being held in Catania, Sicily.

The Palaghiaccio will have all the action.

One hundred and thirteen nations and 937 fencers will be in team and individual events for men and women in épée, foil, and sabre, courtesy of the International Fencing Federation (FIE)—which held the first international championship in Paris in 1921. Italy is currently front and center, but historically the Soviet Union/Russia have won the most gold medals (124), followed by Italy (94) and Hungary (87).

If you want to talk and, in the old days, *see* blood, talk épée. A good attack should net you a point. A lousy one should see your opponent counterattack and demoralize you. But don't feel bad. Way back when, when men were men, and women weren't allowed to play, if you were clumsily aggressive, you'd be a spitted dead duck.

With épée, hesitation kills. At least on points (these days). And don't grip the handle too hard. It's not a vise, rather an instrument for deftness. But if your feet are not properly balanced, with the result that you lack the ability to advance or retreat at will, all your hand, wrist, and arm skills will be for naught, and you will be ripe for the plucking. Foot and hand stamina is a must too, especially if you want to take the gold and the $20,000 that goes with it.

In épée every part of your body is a legitimate target. The sword is an extension of yourself. Mastering attack, defense, and counterattack plus acquiring skills in tactics and strategy is essential—and can take years. Shortcomings, however, can be found out in *milliseconds* because one can double down in épée. That is a double touch that counts if the second touch is within 1/25 of a second of the first.

Oh, and that jolly jumper rope-cord-wire that sends electronic scoring touches to the scorer's box? Not any more, for at Catania now, all weapons are wireless.

Scoring, or at least killing scores of people, has been associated with fencing for quite some time now. Some 20 centuries ago in China, folks looked at fencing as a way to get rid of undesirables. For better or for worse, fencing is now a sport, and it just isn't considered sporting to decapitate an opponent. But it would certainly keep fencing on the front pages following a World Championship.

The sabre ("saber" in American spelling) differs from foil and épée in that the tip - and the edge - of the blade can be used to score.

For sabre, timing is everything. A change to scoring based on touch time differentials threw sport purists for a loop, and tossed technique supposedly into disarray. All hell broke loose. Many derided sabre for decreasing the time differential from 300–350 milliseconds to 120 milliseconds.

The sabre is lightening quick; it is shorter than the foil or épée and lighter than the épée. For the sabre, excluding the hands, any body part from the waist up is fair game. With sabre, green means right and red means left. These lights go on with a scoring touch.

Lights, action, camera. Fencing may have been gruesomely violent at one time, but it's a great job creator. How many extras were employed for the myriad of *Zorro* and *Three Musketeers* movies?

There is a certain panache and élan to fencing, even if the fencing garb and masks, ironically, hide personal mystique. Swinging a thin blade is a magical, delicate, precise act. It's not tossing a caber, all the while praying that a hernia doesn't erupt.

Didn't Robin Hood's swordsmanship rescue Maid Marian?

Don't look for an outsider to rescue you in fencing. It takes inner drive and determination, and adaptation (try matching up against a lefty) to prosper. The drive to thrive comes not so much in competition, but in practice, in repetition. Say you hate a certain attack exercise because you are weak at it. Too bad. You have to practice it anyway. Why? Because you must be able to defend against it.

Fencing is one of just four sports to have been in every modern Olympic Games. Heady enough. What is headier is that, with its requirement for strategy and for disparate physical skills, it is a classic concoction of physicality and brain power.

The Catania 2011 World Fencing Championships was a barometer—in point results—to gauge readiness for the 2012 London Olympics.

Who was on top? In the women's épée, for example, Hungary's Emese Szasz was ranked number one. She won silver in the 2010 World Fencing Championships.

And here's a toughie. Care to guess what the official mascot is for this competition? Give up? Come on down, Fency, for you have been selected. What, or who, is Fency? Fency is a prickly cactus pear. So there.

While Fency may be friendlier than it looks, more than likely it is the 150th anniversary of Italian unification that swung the deal to have Catania, Sicily, as host. That and Italy's illustrious history with fencing.

Fencing has been with us since the times of the Pharaohs. It has evolved from its use in war as a necessity, with horror, to be a chosen instrument in sport, with honor. From killing to keeping score, from rudimentary blades to the finely honed swords of today, one does not need to be an expert to appreciate the finer points of fencing. This dignified sport will continue to delight and excite, and Catania's a great venue.

Chapter 73
Hitting heaven! Roller Derby World Cup 2011

The first Roller Derby World Cup (2011) finished up this past Sunday in Toronto. Fans flocked to the military depot—"The Bunker"—where the bruising sport featured women from 13 countries competing to lay out the opposition on their way to glory, and history.

Since the 1970s, roller derby has sort of been lost like Moses was for his 40 years wandering the desert. But roller derby is back with a gusher of a vengeance, and the ladies have gruesome tattoos and are armed with intestinal fortitude, guts,—guts that guys can only match by drinking 24 beers. The women love this venture precisely because body contact is allowed—heck it's encouraged; more than that, it's essential. This isn't namby-pamby stuff.

Any sport that calls its competitions *bouts*—well, you get the idea. And *Blood and Thunder* is a magazine on all things roller derbyish. So what *is* this roller skating revival of the round, pound all about?

Well, it's as lively as we might expect. Recently, the USA took home the bacon, winning first prize, with Canada second and England third, at the 2011 Roller Derby World Cup. The Derby News Network (DNN) provided the live online coverage. Their reporting on the games, in this case the final game between the USA and Canada, where the Americans stomped the Canadians 336–33, speaks to the sport's gnarly, colorful terminology and colossally wonderful player nicknames:

It was 38–0 there, and Canada got an opportunity when Williams was boxed as jammer for Team USA; however, Disco Akers, Urrk'n Jerk'n, Joy Collision and Frida Beater would not let Canada jammer Smack Daddy find any daylight. Even with a minute in the box, Williams still managed to complete her first pass and add 9–0 to USA's score, and Smack Daddy ended the jam on the box on a major track cut.

Not sure what this means, but then again the writer does not have 10 kids loaded for bear in a Mosh Pit pack mentality, ransacking the house. For sure the play-by-play sounds a heaping less staid than professional golf's, where commentators whisper about a six-foot downhill putt dropping, as "courageous."

Hollywood bravely got onto the roller derby bandwagon with *Whip It*, a story of a young Texas teen who seeks her future in this not genteel, but totally real sport.

She was certainly committed, dropping a life of beauty pageants to follow this extreme dream. Drew Barrymore directed the movie.

Is roller derby headed anywhere? For sure it's headed up, having resurrected itself from decades of decline. You don't get women from wildly disparate cultures and from way-off distant lands like New Zealand, Brazil, France, and Finland, to name but a few vying nations, unless the sport has an overwhelming, unifying theme of crunching competition.

Roller derby had become largely choreographed by the 1960s and '70s, and fans already had professional wrestling to fill that niche, so the sport died. But in 2001, when it started to revive in Austin, Texas, the rebirth was due to the belief that to survive and thrive, it must feature real spills, chills, and thrills. Pain, punishment, power, and precision sell well.

Flat tracks rule the arenas. Over 98% of the 400+ leagues worldwide use this surface (as opposed to a banked track) and it brings the competitor literally, after being hip checked off the track, into your face or onto your lap. Protect that popcorn.

Befitting its authenticity, roller derby has rules. Of course what you are allowed to do boggles the mind, but that's why the more timid and voyeuristic amongst us can be spectators. The do's and don'ts are laid out by the Women's Flat Track Derby Association (WFTDA).

The nuts and bolts of this sport of jolts are made up of 8 blockers and 2 jammers. The jammers have to get past the blockers (the pack) to score. Each blocker passed earns a point. Of course, the blockers will try to shoulder, hip, or booty check the jammer into the next county. But the jammers get through. Don't try elbowing a jammer in the head, blocking from the back, or tripping them at the knee—these are penalties. *Rink rash*—when flesh gets flayed on a rink surface—is perfectly unacceptable, is to be expected, is part of the game, and is completely legal to boot. Ouch. The two periods of 30 minutes each, are pretty well non-stop action.

Even though the sport is insanely physical, sanity dictates the player wear helmet, elbow pads, knee pads, and wrists guards—and skimpy outfits. Oh yeah, the jammers have a large star on their helmets. Jammers are like your football halfbacks or quarterbacks—they take the pounding—but take most of the adulation too.

The USA certainly deserves all the cheers from this inaugural Roller Derby World Cup. Canada scored 9 points to "… make it 105–9—more points than any team had previously managed to score in a game against USA." That pretty well says it all.

Not quite.

For the number-crunching statistics hunter, modern roller derby has three sources of math machinations for your deliberations: WFTDA rankings; Flat Track Stats; DNN Power Rankings. All have come a long way in a short period of time and nicely cover data for competitions, sport skill specifics, and team-by-team assessments. The Derby News Network Power Rankings FAQ has great answers—informative yet irreverent. You can tell the writer(s) love the sport, in and outside the lines of acceptable play, but don't take themselves stuffed-shirt, snob-snot seriously.

But to be seriously ranked and worthy, a combination of good offense and good defense wins. Sound nauseatingly familiar? And while nobody likes to get pasted, the feeling is that the other teams, although below the USA in skill, did have exciting games against teams closer to their level—and that all will be back for the 2012 Roller Derby World Cup.

Chapter 74
Jump at the 2011 Trampoline World Championships

Or, if you missed that one, at the next one that comes your way. Here's what happened in 2011:

Killer moves. Bouncing and bounding our way is the bountiful 2011 Trampoline World Championships.

The event will see the world's best gymnasts in trampoline, tumbling, and double mini trampoline competing in one of the biggie competitions in the International Federation of Gymnastics (FIG) calendar. Metz, France, hosted the 2010 championship meet.

This year's meet, at the NIA in Birmingham, England, encompasses eight events, four each for men and women, from November 17th to 20th, with more than 600 gymnasts from 40 countries taking part. The World Age Group Championships, junior competition, will see approximately 1200 of the best up and coming young gymnasts from around the world competing too.

To watch these twisting, turning, tumbling trampoliners is to wonder: Won't they get motion sickness? As they catapult 20 or so feet into the air, head over toes, arms outstretched, everywhere mixing somersaulting with stiff-as-a-board vaulting, you figure a wipeout is coming—with this jump—no, that jump—no, *that* jump. Then, routine over, you sigh in relief. You realize you've been tensed up, holding your breath.

These artist-acrobats are thin and lithe but *alive and some kind of strong*. It is tempting to think their sport is a soft touch. These air thespians are spring-"boarded" into action right? But that very action creates a whole host of difficulties. It takes lots of muscle resolve to not only perform the designated degree-of-difficulty motions but to avoid soaring off into the wild blue yonder in a flurry of uncontrolled commotion.

The moves are amazing. What's even more amazing is that the sport survives at all when one considers the dreary ever-present reality of social wet blankets who want all of us to take no risk, take no chance, have no fun, do no dance. How can a sport thrive under these confined, careful, cautious, constrictive bubbles of protection? Many meek mice do seek to tramp out trampolining by regulation and fiat.

Seriously. This is how busybodies see it. They want this sport tossed because, well, sometimes youngsters get hurt. There is a method to their madness. Let's call it death of sport by attrition. Here's how it works:

Basically these pettifogs don't want kids taking the sport up, and if the whipper-snappers somehow do, they insist it be only under expert supervision. But how are expert supervisors nurtured? They don't spring out of nature willy-nilly. They must have been kids at some point.

But if kids are winnowed out because the number of experts dwindles over time, boom!, the party's over, there's no sport to spark, and all is gloom, covered in chaff. The future could forecast a dearth of guides and the death of the trampoline. The wusses and sour pusses would have won the war on fun.

In one cool way, trampoline competitions have a near sudden-death element. Unlike gymnastics, where if you fail a move or fall off an apparatus, you can continue—in trampoline events, if you blunder, an "interruption" has occurred—and your routine is over. You're done like dinner, rendered asunder.

Psst—is Australia, the Land Down Under, being underhanded in marketing the near-illicit trampoline to kids? In Sydney, the youngsters can have a 45-minute session with a professional instructor, if there is at least one parent on standby.

There is further hope. Try this on for size: A NASA study found that 10 minutes on the trampoline was equivalent to a 30-minute run. And it is *68% more efficient* as a cardiovascular workout. Amazing, isn't it, that the springy mat makes things obviously cushy but also surprisingly marvy for general fitness.

The mat is a miracle worker. It absorbs 80% of the body weight. It is way easier and better on the joints than is the pound-pound-pound of running around.

No pussyfooting around *these* facts: The last four World Championships (2005, 2007, 2009, and 2010) had either a Russian or Chinese man or woman win. These competitors are perhaps best personified by Dong Dong. His name is unforgettable, and so is his act. He won gold for China in 2009 and 2010 in the individual men's event.

Dong and other elite trampoline acrobats have taken the basic bounce, the tuck, the tuck jump, and the pike, and pulled them up a fair hike. Just how well they have done so is scrutinized carefully by judges who rate and score the execution of moves in a routine, and the degree of difficulty of those moves.

The epitome of the ascent of elementary exertions to an extraordinary culmination is the "killer." Literally. Here's the definition: A double back somersault with four complete twists.

Trampolines sprang into dandy eye-candy hundreds of years ago with the advent of circuses. Circuses, of course, have the big top—just as well—for powerful trampoliners can bound 25 to 30 feet straight up.

With trampolining, there's more than enough to best show your stuff. With boffo sounding moves like the Barani, the Cody, and the Cradle, this sport is the consummate exhibition of freedom from inhibition, and of unshackled performances that push past the very edges of the sport's standards. Sure, there is a myriad and a multitude of maneuvers to learn. Chances are, if one is to master the discipline to competititve levels, one must start young, around nine years of age, when the body and brain are very adaptable and malleable. For sure, we old folks will revel to a new level, gawking and watching the test of the competitors' limits at the Trampoline World Championships 2011.

Chapter 75
IAAF World Race Walking Cup 2012 in Saransk, Russia

The best movers and shakers strutted May 12th–13th, 2012 in Saransk. People have been walking quickly since dinosaur days, but the official World Walking Cup has only kicked in since 1961.

Some, like Ecuadorian Jefferson Perez, married three World Cups (20 kilometres) with a smooth walking style. Others, like Spaniard Jesus Angel Garcia, couldn't separate success from a struggling step—but he is living proof that amazing athletic accomplishments, including many medals in major competitions (save for the Olympics) can come from, or despite, an awkward gait.

Saransk, in the Russian Republic of Mordovia, is home to the National Olympic Race Walking Training Center. 2012 marks Garcia's 9th appearance in IAAF World Championships. And Mr. Longevity (19 years in competition) is also Mr. Consistent Quality: he's always been 14th or better in these World Walking Cups.

Race walking is rigorous and its finishers, like marathon racers, do sometimes fall in a heap at the finish line. As did Kerry Saxby-Junna of Australia, known for her go-for-broke efforts.

Race walking combines the cadence of a 400-metre runner with the staying power of a stamina specialist for 31 miles or 50 kilometres. Or, for those not keen on such a long-winded scene—try the 20-kilometre race walk—with the criterion that no matter the distance, one foot must be on the ground at all times. Otherwise you'll be grounded.

The elite men and women can scoot along at a pace under seven or eight minutes per mile—for a 12-mile race walk. The feet, however, can be quicker than the eye. That can create controversy because judges, not cameras, rule on posture and foot-to-ground contact.

To make haste, scrap waste. With race walking, efficiency in motion and energy spent, as well as excellence in time, essentially result from keeping the foot that is not touching the ground *close to the ground*. A race walker must also try to maintain an upright posture. Failing to do so can hurt the lower back. To avoid terrible strain there—*do not* lean forward or backward.

The North American Racewalking Institute (NARI) leans to philanthropy, and is dedicated to funding kids up to college in their quests to become top-notch race walkers. Actually, "North American" is a bit misleading with respect to funding: right now only US youth can get in on this. But generally, race walking lovers do support their sport, and provide lots of free instructions on how to race walk correctly.

Race walking is not passive: you *do* actively raise the foot off the ground—but not so much as to have your push send you off line or off balance. The body's "motor" is in the pivot of the hips. In a well-trained race walker, a proper forward hip pivot can *add six inches to the stride.*

Women and men both take part in 10 and 20 kilometre races, but because, let's generalize here, men do so little work around the house, the organizers "that be" dictated that men could walk a 50-kilometre race too.

And for the IAAF World Race Walking Cup in Saransk, normal weather conditions wouldn't be too wet or too warm: Competitors could expect 48% humidity with temperatures around 18 degrees Celsius.

Let's raise the temperature and talk turkey about cold hard cash. Race walkers have to lustily love their sport because the prize money is not anything to email (or French kiss) home about. Contestants can get US$30,000 for the win, $15,000 for the place, and $10,000 for the show. At least with that dough they should be able to keep themselves in shoes.

Speaking of those shoes, here are the basics. Don't buy for fashion, buy for fit. If you find the perfect pair, wear 'em only for racing—maybe for training—but that's it. A great shoe does not grow on a tree so don't unnecessarily wear them out.

What of price? Don't buy cheapies—they'll fall apart faster than a Kim Kardashian marriage. And don't go top of the line either, for the priciest shoes won't be amazingly or even appreciably better than a good medium-priced shoe. And don't be enough of a sucker to fall harder for a celebrity-endorsed shoe than Tiger Woods fell from grace.

Some shoes offer stability—which is great for the race walker—but to get the foot rollover needed for (metaphorically) breakneck speeds, a more flexible shoe is best.

Race walking also burns 1.5 to 2 times the calories as easy walking does. And speed is determined, or best increased, *not* by the length of stride, but by the number of strides taken per minute. Top notch walkers hit 200–240 steps every 60 seconds. Swing your arms in short pendulums with elbows bent, in sync with your legs.

The key is learning how to "legally" race walk before working on increased speed and longer distances. Mexican race walkers, for example, have often walked away with both the team and individual awards (1977, 1979, 1993, 1995), by focusing on this approach. Russia is always a power in this heel-and-toe sport, and based on its results individually and in team competition in the 2010 event, was expected to do very well in Saransk, as was China. A record number of athletes from 67 member federations, a record number in itself, was expected for 2012.

And just so you know... the Cup of Lugarno/World Cup is named after Armando Libotte, the first Chairman of the IAAF Committee of Race Walking, who hailed from Lugarno.

All hail the race walkers who rock. You put a Latin salsa beat to those hips in heat, and apart from the intellectual admiration you'll have watching the speeds achieved, more than likely you'll just say: neat. And the IAAF World Race Walking Cup in Saransk, Russia, is where they meet to compete.

Chapter 76
Kalahari Augrabies Extreme Marathon 2011

Wanna be a BIG DADDY? Take six days to tromp, stomp, and romp in the Kalahari Augrabies Extreme Marathon 2011. The Kalahari is a desert that occupies much of southernmost Africa. Still up for it?

The race runs for 250 kilometers. Can *you*?

A thousand questions come to mind. How much insanity is essential for this? (Race rules insist the runners run over the warmest part of the day.) How much fun is involved? Is this fun measured microscopically? Who looks after the family? Will the family be there upon your return? How much money in running shoes do you go through? Does this mean baby goes without diapers? How many of you are running away from life: child support payments, and marriage promises made and marred by a touch of the grape? How many hours of training per day are there? Do you talk to yourself whilst plodding along? Wouldn't it be great if you could save, store, and sell the sweat? Does the winner let it all hang out, showing there's no funny biz, by taking a whiz, to prove they're clean?

What if you run out of water? What if you get lost?

How can a celebration with a winner's trophy come close to offsetting dehydration, exhaustion, frustration, disorientation, starvation, and deprivation?

Plus calculation. With a race of this distance, GPS coordinators are needed and not all days are created equal: day four is the longest haul at 74 kilometres. There are six stages over seven days: there is no day five. Is lounging and lollygagging around, taking a day off, even legal? The days will exceed 40 degrees Celsius, the nights will drop to under five. The race gets off to a rocky start, literally, at Daberas in Northern Cape, South Africa.

Runners needn't overly freak—there are checkpoints every seven kilometres or so, to ensure they don't disappear off the face of the earth. But who keeps the checkpoint folks safe from marauding hyenas and lions?

Besides an unremitting spirit of adventure, necessities would include: water and an eye examination for each eye—because if you *don't* see mirages and oases, you have big problems. Make sure, too, you have at least run a few marathons before undertaking this fit-for-the-undertaking-profession event.

Did you get a physical beforehand? Never mind the mental checkup. Obviously, the mentally crazy do this deal; it's safe to assume they did not get their heads read beforehand. Check for chafing. Don't get bored; don't get gored by a boar.

Seriously, the race has a team of experts that monitors the competitors. Food is inspected pre-race to ensure adequate calories. And there is a catchy official song—rocks and sand and space—it runs for two minutes, 35 seconds.

But don't think prior planning of the route will guarantee perfect performance: the details of each day's trek are given out that very morning.

Why run the KAEM? The answers center on the physical and mental challenge, the off-road racing, the camping under the stars by night, and the seeing and soaking in of the Northern Cape's Green Kalahari beauty and bounty by day.

Besides having the stamina of a daycare employee working a triple shift—the runner, along with attitude and athleticism, must bring compulsory equipment including: knife, food, water, torch, insect net, whistle, sun protection, blister treatment(s), clothing, cooking stuff, sleeping bag—you know, things for survival.

Don't, however, think the race organizers are heartless, oh no, for here's what they kick in: safety pins, a race number, a space blanket and… that's it.

How does one train for an extreme marathon? If you are a city slicker, it will be near impossible to emulate the desert terrain and conditions of the Green Kalahari. It is located in the northwest corner of South Africa, a land beholden to the Orange River that is either lush wine vineyards or semi-arid desert. It is chock full of the aforesaid lions and hyenas, plus well stocked with cheetahs and leopards for good measure.

Can one find the training time for a 26-mile run six days out of seven? Don't even try. The best answer is to mix off-road running into a regular workout regimen, to acclimatize your feet to different surfaces and try and squeeze in three to four runs per week of 30 miles or so, for a few weeks in a row.

Walk. Mix that walking with running—unless you plan to be up with the fleet elite. (It's murder to crank up that body to run again after walking for an extended period of time.)

Don't try to keep up with the Jones's. Run at your own pace. And practice run with a backpack up and down hills, and at night. Do partial leg squats.

Some think running an extreme marathon at a relatively leisurely pace is not so much of a physical or mental strain as a standard marathon at top speed. Maybe. Wonder if the 29 or so participants, 12 from South Africa, would agree…

Take the race in psychological and physical chunks. Run to the check points and tally each such achievement in the success column. And hope the folks there offer encouraging words.

In the end, of course, it isn't the time taken, nor the speed attained throughout, that governs how you'll be judged in the extreme marathon. You, ultimately, are the final arbiter, the final judge, of whether the journey, including the countless runs in training, has been a success. Did the race and the preparation free you from the drudgery of everyday life? Did you push yourself, healthily, to mental and physical heights previously unscaled? Do you still have dreams, eagerly anticipating the next ultra distance race? If so, then yes, this BIG DADDY Kalahari Augrabies Extreme Marathon 2011 has been a success—every step of the way.

Quite a seven days.

Chapter 77
Jellyfish stings Diana Nyad's Xtreme dream swim

When endurance swimmer Diana Nyad's arms wouldn't extend... you do the math.

The 103-mile "Xtreme dream" is now history, paralyzed by a Portuguese Man o' War. Diana certainly added things up: "Later, I learned that 80 percent of open water swims are cancelled because of jellyfish stings, and no swimmer has ever swum past a Man o' War encounter."

It's not like she gave up the ghost. She swam for some *34 hours* after the first attack, but when her EMT Jon Rose suffered anaphylactic shock from a sting *he* got, pulling stingers off her, well—hey—time to call it a day.

Say, can you imagine a training swim session of 12 to 14 hours? Can't? Don't feel bad: Most people can't fathom 12 hours of anything—unless it's a NCIS marathon on TV.

The casual observer, not knowing what Diana's made of, might well ask: Why do this? Why fight sharks, stingrays, salt water, and no light at night for what, the ho-hum 15 minutes of fame?

And the bystander might also imagine swimming in an ocean would be inexpensive. The ocean water is free and plentiful. Bathing caps don't cost more than a few dollars. Flippers are prohibited; there's a few bucks saved.

But you'd be wrong. The first attempt—a 29 hour, 50 mile try—cost *a half million dollars*. But Diana set the record for long distance swimming without a shark cage, 102.5 miles. You'd reckon, cage or no cage, anybody that resilient and resolute would be tough rawhide for any shark to chomp.

Diana is 62. She's no spring chicken, but she's lion-hearted, with King of the Beast goals. She had famous old-timers helping out: She was to sing Janis Joplin, Bob Dylan and Beatles' golden oldies, beat for beat, stroke by stroke, as she battled waves, wildlife, and whatnots, going for broke.

What is it in the human spirit that pushes and prods a person to such prodigious performances? Why hasn't the thrill of such voyages died for Diana? If you've already swum a million miles, give or take, would a million and one be all that different?

Is it curiosity, to test the limits of human capacity for pain, play, prowess, and performance? Or is this simply a love story, a tale of an effervescent woman enraptured by her sport, with a longing that never dulls, dims, or turns to dust?

And must anybody *even try* to top Diana Nyad? God, think of the herculean hours in prep and pep.

Nike has that catchy motto: "There Is No Finish Line" but those are throwaway words compared to Diana's deeds. Forget finish line; *there is no horizon*.

Diana hopes older folks will take her travails and triumphs to heart, and hunker up enough zip to get up and shake a leg themselves. She also hoped this crossing might help bridge the political abyss that divides Cuba from the USA by swimming from Cuba to Florida.

It could never be smooth sailing for Ms. Nyad, *she's asthmatic*. But take a breath and ask yourself this: What on earth would Diana draw upon to think up and take on such a colossal challenge when it was *30 years since she last swam*?

Well, Diana knows her capacity for work. This swim is stamped in her memory, for she planned on counting up those countless hours spent in training.

Despite the half million dollars raised for the first 2011 swim alone, despite the efforts of pulmonary specialist Dr. Michael Levine who had come up with a remedy for another possible asthma attack like the one that sunk her swim a month before, despite finding the right doctor for her languishing left shoulder in Dr. Jo Hannafin (who had a hand in ameliorating a tear in the biceps tendon), despite Dr. Neal Elattrache's counseling to help deter the right shoulder rotator cuff from scraping against a bruised humerus bone, despite the work of her top notch physical therapist, Karen Joubert, and finally, despite a crew that included shark experts, navigators and weather routers' best collective efforts—the Xtreme Dream of some 200,000 strokes and the triumph of touching Florida, came to naught in a blot, a nature bite of supreme, sinister spite.

Thanks a heap, Portuguese Man o' War (a box jellyfish) for stinging Diana, like, everywhere: on both arms, the side of her body, and the face, only one hour into the crossing.

These pernicious Portuguese Man o' Wars may have won a venomous victory of sorts, but Diana's courage in the face of pain is not the sting of defeat, but the ring of reason, of deference to Mother Nature and her unfathomable and unforgettable ways.

Before we in the cheap seats click back to regularly scheduled NFL programming—we should remember one thing, okay, two things:

First, this is not a case of a favorite team being intimidated by the crowd, or being screwed over by the ref. This is a battleground where non-game combatants entered the field of play and its poisonous proceedings.

Second, this is not a game between two sides with equal numbers, but is a match between a sole swimmer (not forgetting her super support team, but you know what we mean) and teeming seas of fearsome watery foes.

Diana Nyad's blog offers the harrowing account.

Robert Browning put it best: "Ah, but a man's reach should exceed his grasp, Or what's a heaven for?" That makes Diana Nyad a star, right?

Cover up her face in shame? Never should she, nor should we cast any blame. Definitely she's achieved a worthy, well-earned fame to go with her persona and—now in the headlines again—name. But one's gotta feel, one's gotta know, that that surely, simply, wasn't Diana Nyad's ultimate game.

Fittingly, on Labor Day of September 2, 2013 Diana, after nearly 53 hours in the ocean, completed the Cuba to Florida swim! The first swimmer ever to do it without using a protective shark cage. It was her fifth attempt to do so. Going forward, the sharks will need cages. Diana rules the waves.

Chapter 78

Keen! Lindsey Vonn, ski racer to 2018!

This piece was written in late 2011. (Time magazine, in 2013, named Lindsey in its icons section as one of the "100 most influential people in the world.")

Things are looking up for American ski racer Lindsey Vonn. Not only is she the first American woman to win in all five disciplines, if she plays her cards right, she could have the most World Cup wins ever—all by the time she reaches 30.

To be sure, at 46 wins, she has a way to go. But Lindsey has nearly blown away the opposition this season, winning 5 of the first 6 races.

Aah, you ask, but isn't competitive ski racing a game for young women (and men)? Won't advancing age work against her? Not so much anymore. Training, nutrition, and coaching have all improved in recent years. Lindsey points to the men's circuit for inspiration and to her own body, which feels just fine, thank you, even after 11 years on the circuit.

She scaled new heights, finally winning a giant slalom (GS) at Soelden in the first race of the year and now she can tackle the slalom, her weakest link. Hey—she then won another giant slalom at Lake Louise and she wants to use those GS wins as a confidence-builder. It may seem odd to talk confidence when talking Lindsey Vonn, but even a supreme athlete's confidence is as fleeting as a downhill run.

Looking at ski racing from the safety of a reclining lazy-boy, armed with nothing more than a remote, is still a nerve-tingling, jaw-clenching, experience. The slope angles of the ski hill confound: As the cameras track skier progress around tight curves, it seems those athletes will ski off the end of the earth—for gravity alone won't be enough to restrain their momentum into the solar system. They shush down the hill at what, 50 some miles per hour? And that is for the GS. Downhill speeds can hit over 70 mph.

How can skiers spot indentations and best lines on the mountain when the sky is slate gray under a blizzard? And, darn it, minutes earlier the conditions promised bright, clear, sunny sailing. Before the next bend, the racer must view, collate, and calculate the changing hill conditions. This isn't tennis where an all points bulletin goes out at the sniff of showers. How do Lindsey and her ilk react calmly when the weather, acting as though it were nature or something, changes uncontrollably?

It's hard to fathom how a skier can excel at five disciplines all calling, for special requirements in physical skills and specific equipment. The super giant slalom, or super G, and the downhill are known as speed events, the slalom and giant slalom as technical ones. Please don't ask what the fifth discipline, the super combined, entails. The difference between being Queen of the Hill and runner up can be, even for the super G, 1/100th of a second. That's a blink of an eye, right?

Lindsey Vonn, with her twinkling eyes, beaming smile, and sunny disposition, adds a lively light and insight to any interview, in English or in German. She's 27. She knows *exactly* where she wants to go with her skiing career even if, like most of us in our professions, she wants to learn from her mistakes without unduly harping on them. There's a fine line between introspection and depressive navel-gazing, especially when the margins—from excellence to error—are razor thin. She's determined to find the right balance to ensure her poor finishes in the slalom at the end of last season don't happen again.

Reading Lindsey's tweets, first talking about a great training run and then talking about winning the following race, one can only admire the uncanny connection she can make between potential and performance, and enthuse about how she puts both into practice.

Want to test your muscular endurance and general balance? Try holding the skier's crouch for two to three minutes. Now try it while going down a hill steeper than sin. Even watching Lindsey Vonn in a slalom training run, with turns every second or so, shows the core and lower body strength needed for such grueling, exacting exertions.

What attitudes are needed to excel in ski racing? Perspective and patience. Lindsey Vonn did not finish in her December 18, 2011, race in Courchevel. She's not pleased—but she's not *down*. And her homespun philosophy serves her well too: "When you fall down, just get up again."

But it's her bravery, her willingness to dare, her go-for-it gumption to adopt new methods that sealed the deal in making her *the top female skier worldwide*.

Lindsey, at 20, turned her ski training and fitness routines upside down. Overhauling all, she joined forces with Coach Robert Trenkwalder. Her high altitude athleticism peaked—but at first she must have seriously wondered about the risks she was taking in messing with a good thing. A comparable athlete might be Tiger Woods changing his swing when at the top of his game.

To be malleable and not deem oneself infallible due to stellar skiing success is surely integral to staying on top. Bouncing back after being flattened by injury is essential. Persistence, despite race result resistance, is surely crucial too. Lindsey "Don Don" Vonn, chock full of these features, is also capable of rigorous self-analysis, focusing on her progress and position—unvarnished by praise, prejudiced or otherwise, from family and friends. This trait, it must be said, also separates Lindsey from some of the competition. She's world famous, the best female American ski racer ever, and should she continue apace she'll one day be alone, on the throne, in the rarefied air of a professional champion nearing perfection. With her will on the hill, she'll be ruler of the skiing citadel.

Wait…great, this in, of late! She hopes to end her racing reign after the 2018 Winter Olympics in Pyeongchang, South Korea.

(But first, Lindsey who, in 2013, tore two ligaments in her right knee, doesn't know if she'll be able to compete in the Winter Olympics in Sochi, Russia in 2014.)

Chapter 79
Felicity Aston skis across Antarctica solo!

Did you know felicity comes from skiing across Antarctica alone? Felicity Aston does. She not only set a world record for this amazing feat in 2012, she did it knowing first-hand how formidable that frontier is. She'd worked there as a meteorologist.

At first, it's hard to grasp the significance of the fact that she was alone. Countries send down teams for this or that purpose, and are so pleased with themselves, making sure that all their brave-and-batty forays are televised.

But 34-year-old British skier Felicity did this on her lonesome and—okay, so why?

Before we wonder why any further, let's look at the "whats." She not only took herself on this trip, she pulled two sledges.

For 1,084 miles (1,744 kilometers).

Whether reckoned in metric or imperial measure, this unreal crossing—hold it!—isn't it either damn dark or glaringly bright down there, 25 hours out of every day, eight days a week? How did she battle lunacy and loneliness, facing whiteouts, katabatic winds, and fierce sun? Well, the music of Junip and Ben Howard helped.

While she's not a penguin, she's a tough bird nonetheless. She did a marathon in the Sahara (Southern Morocco), led expeditions in Greenland, the Arctic, and Antarctica, and rooted out herbs in Siberia—but this was a one-woman slog among mountains and crevasses between Leverett Glacier and Hercules Inlet. She did have a few companions: cranky knees, sore fingers, and "frost nibbled lips."

Let's give lip service to the math. The trek took 59 days (and 63 phone casts). Fair enough. She had to eat, right? She's fit, not fat, so she couldn't live off her own blubber. She'd need tons, well anyway, lots of sustenance to keep her energy up and to keep from freezing—so let's assume three squares per day.

59 x 3 = 177 meals. Must we therefore conclude that she ate grist, mist, or sawdust? Most of us have a hard time balancing the pizza taken from fridge to table. How could she lug 177 meals with all the fixings of protein, carbohydrates, and the "good" fats? She did have two food drop-offs, which reduced the weight she had to take with her. Oh yeah, but she's gotta drink too. Liquid is heavy. Let's assume she

didn't cart red wine with her. But what of tea and milk? (Water, even if in a snowy, icy form, could be readily had. Might have to be warmed up though...)

For a last meal, she supped on beef and ale stew.

Felicity didn't stew, but being an accomplished travel writer, detailed in her blog how she learned to cope with loneliness and homesickness—by looking at the stars. Her mother told her, when Felicity was around 10, to look up at the sky and know that she was looking at the same sky too. That's a good tip.

And here's another. Felicity trekked in the summertime. Though she talks of 30-degree days, temperatures are generally not bone-chilling killing, coming in at the McMurdo station at a hot and heavy 3 degrees Celsius daily average. And the place is lit more than Charlie Sheen on a bender.

Now, how about that battle against lunacy? This isn't some crazy joke being waged at her expense: She writes of the risk of loony behavior due to *hypothermia*, a potentially fatal drop in body temperature. No biggie there, that would be par for this course, no? Hypothermia can trigger insanity, resulting in actions contrary to one's well-being. For instance people who are freezing to death may actually remove clothing, thinking they are too hot!

Felicity (and other experts) know that the trick to nipping hypothermia and erratic actions in the bud is to have a bud, a buddy, another crew member on hand, to let you know you're slipping off the deep end.

But she was *alone*. Who was to be her early warning wacko alarm? She relied on heavy doses of common sense. Methodically, she'd ask herself: Was a change in plan precipitated by boredom or exhaustion at the end of the day, or was it instilled as a rational thought made when energy and mental focus was high?

(But she rightly freaked when her lighter failed her and she had *just 46 matches left.*)

Felicity travelled as light as possible. The two sledges carried her fuel, Fuizion freeze-dried food, a pot of peanut butter, layered and breathable clothing, and equipment. The overriding rule was that a gram of anything not absolutely needed was not taken. Her two little stoves could be held in the palm of each hand.

She trained diligently and could be seen dragging two car tires on pavement via a rope harness. She took solace from her followers via social media and sustenance from her sponsor, Kaspersky Labs. Her groundbreaking trip was called Kaspersky ONE Transantarctic Expedition 2011.

When she speaks to kids of her exploits, she uses terms everyone can all shake, quake, and relate to. The air outside on such a trip would be *twice as cold* as your freezer at home.

To bear those unbearable temperatures, to last, and to live, Felicity focused on stamina, doing low intensity workouts and eschewing a he-woman, big-muscle complex. Upper thighs (for skiing) and shoulder blades (for pulling) bore the brunt of her resistance training.

But now, journey finished, the luxury of hot water showers, wine, company, and the plaudits of worldwide press coverage via CNN and British newspapers naturally follow. She's up in spirits and down in weight. Judging from Felicity's accounts on Twitter, she seems remarkably level-headed and chipper. About the only down-side to this dénouement is the downer her 9,400+ Twitter followers may feel, not hearing the latest from this intrepid explorer and her unreal expedition in the vast icy, dicey landscape *way down under.*

They can, however, read all in her new book: Alone in Antarctica!

Chapter 80

Felix Baumgartner's space jump goose bumps

This piece was written before Felix's record breaking skydive of October, 2012.

Everybody should do a mission to the edge of space and then bail from a height of 120,000 feet if they are tired of their current conditioning program.

No?

Okay, let's leave the high-flying, diving act to Felix Baumgartner.

And yes, you read that correctly—120,000 feet. That's about three times the cruising height of your basic passenger jet; they go a paltry eight miles up. Baumgartner's ballooning 23 miles up. Gulp. Why would Felix do this? He says he's curious…

More on Felix Baumgartner in a jiffy.

Who else benefits? Medical director Dr. Jonathan Clark. He is currently with the National Space Biomedical Research Institute. He was the crew surgeon for six space shuttle flights. He has been chomping at the bit to research and record how a space, cadet fall like this one might help space tourism.

Who lives? Possibly Felix Baumgartner. And, more likely, anybody who doesn't try this.

This free fall or plummet, call it what you will, certainly won't be free. Red Bull is the sponsor; the money's got to come from somewhere. The ground team (seven in all) probably get paid on a "galaxy and a half" basis. Everything's gotta cost.

Felix Baumgartner comes by a love for all-things-sky honestly. He globe-trots around the world more than UN diplomats. He is a helicopter pilot. He's a sky diver. He's a world-record BASE jumper (that is, someone who jumps off buildings, antennas, spans (bridges), and earth (cliffs), breaking his fall with a parachute. But this foray, as he puts it, to *the edge of space,* seems crazy. Parts might be a ball; dropping head first, straight down (the Delta position) might be fun in theory, and in reality. With reduced drag and better stability, the chance to break the speed of sound is improved. After the Delta phase, if all goes well and swell, his parachute will open.

Still, why does an enterprising bloke who has everything to live for want to tempt fate with this feat? And death would hardly be the worst part, it would be the path to that death that would be unbelievably macabre. Without going into all the geek science techno talk, here's what could happen. (All this in particular disorder.)

He could suffer from terminal lack of confidence: What if he misses the Earth and lands, like, nowhere? But let's assume he has a map and is headed straight for us—what might happen on the descent if things go bust? If his space suit develops a hole, he could die in a flash. And with the air pressure up there thinner than China's commitment to human rights, his blood could literally boil. That can't be good for the old allowable body temperature range. Or he might suffocate from a lack of oxygen. Or catch a cold because temperatures hover around 70 to 80 degrees below 0 Celsius.

Also, do you remember learning about the sound barrier in that science class you forgot to cut? Well it's still there, and Felix hopes to cut through it. But this just isn't an amenable stroll through a county boundary where the only risk is running into a yokel sheriff; triggering this out-in-the-wild-blue-yonder sound barrier causes a sonic boom. If his helmet malfunctions, it could be his ears will be cauliflowers and his brain a peanut, or a pizza.

We humans tromp in the troposphere. Felix will soar to the next layer up, the stratosphere. This is heady stuff. But what seems even more incredible is that 52 years ago—52 years ago, without the technological breakthroughs and accumulated scientific knowledge we have today—Col. Joe Kittinger decided he had better go make a freefall from 102,900 feet. Kittinger later remarked about the disorientation and the unfamiliarity of it all, saying he wasn't even sure he was *falling*.

Now it's true that the sound barrier was broken by Chuck Yeager in 1947. But he was in a *plane*. Baumgartner will be in a capsule, then naked except for his pressurized, fire-retardant, insulated astronaut suit.

Currently Baumgartner and his crew are feverishly tying up loose ends at their Roswell, New Mexico, training grounds for the Red Bull Stratos Mission. They successfully launched two unmanned balloon launches. (No word of how the balloons fared on his blog post.) Pressure tests were conducted at the Brooks Air Force Base near San Antonio, Texas.

Hey, wonder if he'll be posting "this just in" updates to his blog if he pulls this off? He has done updates before while high in the sky. Nah—he's got a 12-pound chest pack that will see to that job, sending—in real time—lotsa data to mission control.

Space jumping—Red Bull-style—gotta be an extreme sport, right? It's definitely an extreme sashay. And the 41-year-old Austrian, who has been jumping from ungodly heights since he was a sweet 16, wouldn't have it any other way.

So what happened? The world waited to see how it would play out…

October 14th, 2012 was the day…

The only thing faster than Felix's *843 miles per hour* plummet was the speed at which Cypriots on the financially flattened island of Cyprus did a run on the ATMs before their savings were nearly confiscated by the government.

For sure his core and mental toughness is unparalleled. Apparently, during his descent, for a time he was spinning 60 revolutions per minute, or one per second.

Wait a second.

Let's leave the extreme exercise to this champion space cadet, huh?

The world's voyeurs and scientists will get an emotional and rational buzz out of Felix Baumgartner's 2012 supersonic jump. For Felix the guinea pig, other than the obligatory 15 minutes of fame and an in-the-know soul glow that comes from proving that a human can break the sound barrier, he has to also know that this is a puny return for betting his life.

Chapter 81
Exhort the sport of wife carrying!

How momentous this is. Words can't describe it. "Jaw-dropping" feels like a cliché, but hey, we gotta start somewhere. The sport of wife carrying is here to stay.

This makes eminent sense. One could not have "husband carrying" as a sport because wives carry their husbands in real life, what with chores, kids, playing nursemaid to hubby… There is no sense in staging this fact of life. Who'd watch it?

But wife carrying—well, this is a sport of a different sort—and it is growing by leaps and bounds, or at least as fast as men can man up and get themselves some wives.

Here are the happy facts. As luck would have it, the sport's genesis has its roots in its nemesis, *wife stealing*. Way back, when men used to look around, frustrated that the sticks wouldn't ignite, itching for a fight, tired of scrawling stupid horses in clammy caves in the dark of the night, they'd say—hey, think I need a new wife *today*. And off they'd go a-marauding and a-pillaging, a-hooting and a-hollering, and all this before booze mind you, and ransack a fanny pack in the form of a brand new spouse from the village afar or the neighbor's house—whichever was easier. And thus this necessity, this basic building block of existence so essential to one's lifeblood, levity, and lunacy became a litmus test of all that was good with the world.

Some of the above may be a tad-to-a-ton apocryphal, but the sport had to come from somewhere. Stuff doesn't just pop out of thin air, right?

As it turns out, the sport began in the land of hot air saunas and cold air masses, Finland. A rogue known as Ronkainen the Robber is credited with discovering and popularizing this dynamic, not to be topped, pastime, still followed today.

The rules are, as in any real marriage, hazy, subject to change willy-nilly, and open to interpretation and deliberation—but this much is clear: If the wife is a tomboy and the husband is a nancy-boy, the woman can carry the man. And how one transports another is up to the couple. Piggyback and the fireman's lift are common, but the best means to portage the better half, experts say, is the Estonian lift.

Estonia was known, along with Latvia and Lithuania, for creating the Baltic Way—a human chain of two million people that publicized their wont to escape the claws of the great, grumpy, grabby bear, the old USSR—but this Estonian lift forever etches Estonia on the global map of earth-shattering marital events.

The Estonian lift works like this: Have the wife wrap her arms around hubby's waist. (Let's hope the hubby isn't a fatty but if he is, they probably aren't racing anyway, so let's continue.) Then, somehow or other, make the little woman's legs wind around the shoulders and head of the beleaguered, besieged man. Think of 69 without the sex, one would guess.

And so on they go, these duos, carrying themselves into berths of dirt, over mountains of madness, and streams of sadness. These are married couples imitating life after all, and the winners get, well, if the event was the North American Wife Carrying Championships, for all their troubles and travails, some beer and cash. For those that haven't left this article to practice up—the 2011 winners were Rocco Andreozzi and Kim Wasco, in a mind-numbing, my-aren't-we-humming time of 49.64 seconds. No slumming from this Maine couple, huh?

If motivated and not bummin', with the load not too heavy, a man can run faster than a trot, but not often. Brains, if the woman has some, must be protected by a helmet.

Oh, this just in. The Estonian lift has the *woman's head at the rear of the man*, not the front. Think not the 69 without the sex, just think of the Estonian lift. It's easier. Cleaner. Unless it isn't.

It's hard to say who has the tougher job, the slogging husband or the uncomfortable, hang-on-for-dear, … what-IS-this-kind-of life, wife. Maybe it's one of those kinds of things that makes you stronger if it doesn't annoy you and pester you to death. Who knows, love may even grow.

As befits such a highly technical sport, there are rules. The wife must not be a waif weighing less than 107.8 pounds. If she is, the powers that oversee these exhibitions of marital fidelity fitness load the pair with a bag of lead, or something heavy anyway. Another rule is that the contestants enjoy themselves. That is superfluous. Any couple that likes carrying one another uphill and down dale probably gets excited watching paint dry. For sure, they're going to like this escapade charade.

With video games, Facebook, secret chat rooms, hatred, the puppy, and even those infernal kids taking precious time from spouses' togetherness, it's lovely that wife carrying can bring Jack and Jill back together again. Too often anomie and rampant individuality replace commonality and frivolity. This sport, this event, this way of life, this means to *live*—counterbalances all bothersome, unneeded diversions and acts as the glue that can keep any two together, until death do them part, or until the sport of wife throwing is invented.

Conclusion
Obesity myths dead and buried

One of the biggest problems many of us have in our quest to lose weight is the tsunami of contradictory evidence and studies relating to obesity and fitness. We don't know where to turn or who to believe.

Witness…

In a recent article titled "Doctors Attack Pervasive Obesity Myths," columnist Christopher Wanjek, of *LiveScience* Bad Medicine, points out a few humongous misconceptions most of us (apparently) have about obesity.

We'd like to think that physical education at school would help stem obesity amongst our offspring. We'd expect to think that losing weight quickly is not as good for you as losing weight gradually. We'd dream to believe that we burn oodles of calories fooling around between the sheets. But these three examples of commonplace assumptions are wrong, according to the University of Alabama's David Allison.

It's more than disconcerting to have your beliefs, grounded in previous studies and common wisdom in the right ways to losing weight, be swept away beneath your feet by the latest unassailable research—it's utterly vexing. What's the point of trying this or that, if all that you attempt will be debunked as junk in the next slew of studies to come down the line?

Yet through this entire miasma of conflicting viewpoints, what choice does anyone have but to try to exercise, even if for just 15 minutes per day, and to cut back on junk food? True, there have been studies done showing the benefits accrued from extra physical activity taper off with increased loads of that activity. But nobody, nowhere, to my knowledge has come out and flatly said *any* exercise is bad for you. If such a peer-reviewed study is published, with the science declared unalterably "proven," let's make sure we see who funded the work, what the parameters of that work were, and how the data was manipulated, before we throw in the towel.

There is, however, one obesity myth that we might all like to know is so much bunkum, and that is this: the belief that setting "realistic" rather than colossal weight loss goals is the way to achieve success. Well, according to Allison, data suggests that people do better with more ambitious goals. "Think big to lose big." Go big with your targets or stay home is the message here.

Now let's get under the covers and dangle with the sex angle. Folklore says that a single stint of sultry sex will burn off 300 calories per partner. But if one partner is doing most of the work, this seems unlikely. And if we factor in that the average time of the tryst is just this: six lousy (maybe lustful) minutes then, at most, the calories expended would amount to, the article says, *20*.

Nevertheless, the vast majority of us would rather lose those 20 calories through a carnal coupling than by jogging the same amount of time around the old high school track, unless you're married or something.

Oops, got a bit off base…

Now let's take a look at another so-called "unproven" myth that is certain to upset some apple carts. The jury, apparently, is still out on whether having a healthy breakfast is crucial in the goal of keeping the weight down. Holy cow. All I can draw upon is personal experience when I say that my breakfasts are a major reason why I am not hungry at night. I don't need junk food or whatever else is handy after 7 pm. It makes intuitive sense that eating more earlier in the day would result in less of a need or even an appetite to eat more at night.

Whether a person gains weight ultimately comes down to whether they ingest more calories than they burn. The theory that eating a good breakfast helps weight loss is based on the assumption that the dieter will be active during the day, and expend the calories, and *not* ingest more calories than needed later that night. Seen from that perspective, the big breakfast theory holds true. It is a way of assigning more calories to the part of day when more activity is expected. But it is not a magic formula.

In the final analysis, no matter what pundit A says, or professional B avers, you can tell if exercise and healthier eating is working. As Method Three proves, weight can start coming off from Day One—and continue that way for days on end. And if you are still hitting personal bests in your fitness or sports activities, then you have ample proof that you are more conditioned and capable, and that the foods you have chosen, and their portions and percentages, are working well to support your new athletic achievements.

Well what do we know? We know that if you are a minority, rich or poor, young, middle-aged or old, female or male, or an only child, there's a pretty darn good chance you'll end up overweight or obese. But it doesn't have to be that way. As the four Methods in this book show, there *are options* to either stem an increase in body fat, reduce it, or never pile it on in the first place.

The key, however, is you. Only you can decide to adopt one of these methods or use other strategies, wholly or partly, in reaching your fitness and health goals. Yes, family and friends may encourage you (or harass you to smithereens) but the potential and the power to become what you want to be, at least physically, resides within yourself.

The constants that I found to work, through all four Methods, were walking, using an Elliptical machine, weight training, and keeping track of progress. But above all, the main thing is to have a goal, not a wish. Wishes are too airy fairy, too inconsequential. You must have desire. Whether the motivation underlying that desire is health concerns or simple vanity, your motivation doesn't matter as much as your drive and determination.

It's up to you.

Now get out there and lose.

And gain your life back!

www.ingramcontent.com/pod-product-compliance
Lightning Source LLC
Chambersburg PA
CBHW030309290526
45785CB00001B/269